Recovery, Mental Health and Inequality

T0386184

Mental health has long been perceived as a taboo subject in the UK, so much so that mental health services have been marginalised within health and social care. There is even more serious neglect of the specific issues faced by different ethnic minorities.

This book uses the rich narratives of the recovery journeys of Chinese mental health service users in the UK – a perceived 'hard-to-reach group' and largely invisible in mental health literature – to illustrate the myriad ways that social inequalities such as class, ethnicity and gender contribute to service users' distress and mental ill-health, as well as shape their subsequent recovery journeys.

Recovery, Mental Health and Inequality contributes to the debate about the implementation of 'recovery approach' in mental health services and demonstrates the importance of tackling structural inequalities in facilitating meaningful recovery. This timely book would benefit practitioners and students in various fields, such as nurses, social workers and mental health postgraduate trainees.

Lynn Tang is Assistant Professor in the School of Arts and Humanities, Tung Wah College, Hong Kong.

Routledge Studies in the Sociology of Health and Illness

Recovery, Mental Health and Inequality

Chinese Ethnic Minorities as
Mental Health Service Users

Lynn Tang

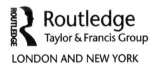

LONDON AND NEW YORK

First published 2017 by Routledge

2 Park Square, Milton Park, Abingdon, Oxfordshire OX14 4RN
52 Vanderbilt Avenue, New York, NY 10017

Routledge is an imprint of the Taylor & Francis Group, an informa business

First issued in paperback 2019

British Library Cataloguing-in-Publication Data
A catalogue record for this book is available from the British Library

Library of Congress Cataloging in Publication Data
Names: Tang, Lynn, author.
Title: Recovery, mental health and inequality : Chinese ethnic minorities as
mental health service users / Lynn Tang.
Other titles: Routledge studies in the sociology of health and illness.
Description: Abingdon, Oxon ; New York, NY : Routledge, 2017. |
    Series: Routledge studies in the sociology of health and illness |
    Includes bibliographical references and index.
Identifiers: LCCN 2017002012| ISBN 9781138849976 (hardback) |
    ISBN 9781315725086 (ebook)
Subjects: | MESH: Mental Disorders—therapy | Asian Continental
    Ancestry Group—psychology | Mental Health Services—organization
    & administration | Ethnic Groups—psychology | Minority Groups—
    psychology | United Kingdom—ethnology | China—ethnology
Classification: LCC RC455.4.E8 | NLM WA 305 FA1 | DDC 362.2089—dc23
LC record available at https://lccn.loc.gov/2017002012

ISBN: 978-1-138-84997-6 (hbk)
ISBN: 978-0-367-22443-1 (pbk)

Typeset in Times New Roman
by Swales & Willis Ltd, Exeter, Devon, UK

Contents

Tables

Acknowledgements

This book is an outcome of my academic, as well as personal, journey to date. It also constitutes the journeys of my research participants. For this journey to be realised, I have the Overseas Research Students Awards Scheme and the Warwick Postgraduate Research Studentship to thank for the full scholarship to pursue the PhD research that this book is based on, as well as the British Sociological Association for the Phil Strong Memorial Prize, which enabled the participants to share their recovery journeys with me. Thanks also go to Amy Cui from the Chinese Community Centre Birmingham, Louise Wong from the Wai Yin Chinese Women Society, as well as Perry Fung and Khim Wong from the Chinese Mental Health Association for their generous help in introducing me to the participants. My deepest gratitude goes to the research participants. I feel honoured to listen to their stories and am touched by their sorrows and strengths in their recovery journeys. I hope this book does justice to their stories.

I must thank my supervisors, Mick Carpenter and Peter Ratcliffe, for persistently raising the bar and widening my academic horizons. Gratitude is extended to David Pilgrim and Hilary Marland for their critical comments on the PhD thesis, and to Bob Carter for his encouragement during the Prato Writing Workshop. I am also thankful to Simon Clarke, Phil Mizen, Joy Fillingham and Mandy Lugsdin for their generous hospitality when I travelled between Hong Kong and the UK; as well as Miu Chan and Kender Wu for their assistance in the research.

Having worked in 'Mental Health in Higher Education', a multidisciplinary teaching and learning project, this broadened my understanding of the contested nature of mental health (problems) as well as the vital role of the service user movement in advancing our knowledge about mental health. I learnt a lot from my wonderful and supportive colleagues Jill Anderson and Hilary Burgess, and would like to thank the Centre of Excellence in Interdisciplinary Mental Health at the University of Birmingham for appointing me as an honorary fellow and offering continuous support during my PhD years.

I am blessed with friendships that provide a solid foundation for me to take on this project. Thanks are due to Charlene Clempson, Anne Barrett, Sarra Facey, Jill Anderson, Jan Wallcraft, Elisabeth Simbürger, Rosario Undurraga, Milena Kremacova, Kirsty Liddiard, Kirsty Warren, Ruth Pearce, Mark Carrigan, Elizabeth Matka, Amalia Schnier, Wai-Ha Lam, Anita Liu, Yubin Chiu, Huamei

Chiu, Debora Poon, Garyin Tsang, Lai Ching Leung, Florence Hui and Mei Tse. Special love goes to Ann Davis and Alex Davis for their enormous faith in me and generous support in myriad forms. I wish Wai-Ling could read this book as she has always been a key part of this journey. I must also thank my dear parents for having always shown unreserved support in my academic pursuit. My profound love is dedicated to Chris King-Chi Chan, my partner, for always being there to share the adventures of life, through better or worse.

1 What recovery? Whose recovery?

Recovery as a disputed approach

Introduction

This book critically interrogates the concept of recovery and the elements of the recovery approach, through exploring the way social inequalities shape the journeys of Chinese mental health service users in the UK. Recovery as a movement originating in the US has gained impetus internationally and has been adopted as a mental health policy paradigm in many different countries (Ramon *et al.*, 2009; Slade *et al.*, 2012). In the UK it has been a frequent discursive feature of policy documents and has been adopted by governments as their 'vision' of mental health services (DoH, 2001, 2009, 2011).

The recovery movement has its roots in new social movements and has concerned itself with asserting the rights of mental health service users to control their own lives in the face of the dominance of psychiatric power. However, criticism had been made of the way recovery has been mainstreamed and appropriated by mental health policies. Such criticism questions the extent that social-structural inequalities leading to, and resulting from, distress and mental ill health, can be addressed in a neo-liberal political economy and policy context (Pilgrim, 2008; Spandler and Calton, 2009; Edgley *et al.*, 2012; Morrow, 2013).

It is against this background that this book aims to problematise the concept of recovery and argue for the central role of social justice at the heart of a recovery paradigm – one that addresses and tackles multilevel inequalities. It aims to achieve this empirically by exploring the lived experiences of a marginalised group of mental health service users. Incepted from my experiences as a Hong Kong Chinese woman who has used mental health services in both the Hong Kong and UK, this book is based on my doctoral research on Chinese service users living in the UK, which illuminates how structural inequalities contribute to their ill health and shape the social conditions in which they recover. This study privileges service user knowledge and illustrates their agency throughout the recovery journeys. Through understanding their struggles of recovery, this book will shed light on the cultural as well as structural factors that facilitates or hinders recovery in a multicultural society for this ethnic minority community.

What recovery?

The first question to be asked about the concept of recovery is, 'What do people recover from?' Recovery as a proposed new paradigm in the philosophy, management, and delivery of mental health services suggests a change from the dominant, pessimistic view of the possibility of recovery from severe mental health illness. Since Kraepelin (1919) formulated the concept of schizophrenia, the bio-medical classification with its pessimistic prognosis has been widely adopted, despite evidence suggesting more optimistic recovery rates (e.g. Warner, 1994; Harrison *et al.*, 2001). Service users receiving a diagnosis of severe mental illness, e.g. recurrent psychotic episodes, are often told they will never be free from psychosis (e.g. Clark, 2007). It is proposed that a recovery approach can move from this notion of chronicity and deficit to therapeutic optimism (Allott *et al.*, 2002; Lester and Gask, 2006; Ramon *et al.*, 2007). Instead of cure and a return to the pre-illness state, Anthony (1993) argues that recovery should be a way of living a meaningful life even with the limitations caused by distress and mental ill health. Therefore, recovery is about social inclusion, being accepted as part of society (Repper and Perkins, 2003). Some service users argue that recovery is a process in which a new life purpose is usually developed (e.g. Deegan, 1988; Clark, 2007). This is a self-defined route of recovery with real choices about accepting or rejecting certain treatment options, including the choice to define recovery in your own way (Coleman, 2004). Spandler and Calton (2009) argue that the dominant recovery discourse being mainstreamed into the mental health policies 'fails to question the dominant ideas about what people have recovery "*from*", whilst social inclusion has no critique of that which people are supposed to be included "*in*"' (p. 251, my emphasis).

Despite the potential of the recovery approach for empowering service users to achieve quality lives, its implementation in different countries has been criticised for its limitations. For example, its individualistic tendency and its lack of a commitment to tackle the inequalities mental health service users face. These limitations, as Morrow (2013) highlights in a critique of the recovery paradigm in Canada, can be traced to the political economical context in which health and social policies are formulated and embedded. Mental health services and policies do not take forms incompatible with neo-liberal logic. The version of the recovery approach that has been mainstreamed lacks the progressive power to challenge the social determinants of mental ill health, including the inequalities upheld by neo-liberalism that contribute to distress. Those elements that aim to tackle inequalities, including existing power inequalities, tend to be marginalised in the mainstream recovery paradigm. This is in spite of the literature that evidences the impact of social determinants on mental health inequity (Weisser *et al.*, 2011).

This same critique is applicable to the context of the UK. Carpenter (2009a) points out that the New Labour changes to the English and Welsh mental health legislation saw an increase in the control of service users and a reduction in their rights. This is contrary to the ethos of self-determination in the recovery approach. As Pilgrim indicates, the growth of consumerism in health care services appropriates some of the service user movements' claims for choice and rights (Pilgrim, 2008), but it has increasingly moved away from the participatory version of choice that the service user movements envision. Services that were effective in promoting social inclusion for service users, for example, day centres, have been closed down in England by the Coalition and the subsequent Conservative government in the name of austerity. Such closures serve to reduce the choices of services users. The government's cut on disability benefits and concerted moral attack on disability claimants, amplified by the demonising discourses of the tabloids, has fuelled the dominant paternalistic, narrow definition or outcome of recovery and social inclusion, which means recovery to work. Harper and Speed (2012) and Rose (2014) warn that the mainstreamed recovery discourse has lost the liberatory and emancipatory element originally proposed in the recovery movement. As recovery is increasingly experienced as a disciplinary force to urge service users to get paid employment and mask persisting coercion, e.g. community treatment order, service user advocates become critical to the recovery discourse, with some even propose an abandonment of the rhetoric of recovery (Pilgrim and McCranie, 2013; Recovery in the Bin, 2016).

Pilgrim (2008) delineates three competing versions of the recovery approach, which are helpful in explicating what the recovery of service users means and entails, and why these meanings may contradict each other. The three meanings of recovery include 'recovery from illness, i.e. an outcome of successful treatment', 'recovery from impairment, i.e. an outcome of successful rehabilitation' with an emphasis on obtaining social skills and 'recovery from invalidation, i.e. an outcome of successful survival' (Pilgrim, 2008: 29). These three meanings can serve as ideal types of recovery discourses in exploring what the recovery paradigm for mental health services is. They can co-exist with each other, for example, in understanding the bio-medical model and the social model of mental health care as 'complementary and synergistic' as outlined in the joint position paper of the Care Services Improvement Partnership (CSIP), Royal College of Psychiatrists (RCPsych) and the Social Care Institute for Excellence (SCIE) (2007: 2). They can also be in tension with each other. For example, the second discourse which promotes the building of social skills that are fit for society could conflict with the third discourse which promotes the reclaiming of full citizenship and freedom from potentially coercive services and self-determination in life choices (Pilgrim, 2008). Such tensions are predicated upon a contradictory feature of mental health services: individual user's choice and risk reduction to serve the public interest, with the latter exemplified in the 2007 Mental Health Act (Carpenter, 2009a). The power to declare recovery resides in mental health professionals to whom the state confers powers to exercise coercive social control. This conflicts with users' choices to be service avoiders, rejecting the notion that mental distress is an illness or choosing to live lives that deviate from social norms. The first and second discourses adopted by mental health services and main professional bodies, mask the imperative to change oppressive and excluding social structures that can invalidate service users, an imperative that is central to the third discourse.

A sociological understanding of the interplay of structure and agency helps take the question of 'What is recovery?' further (G.H. Williams, 2003; S.J. Williams, 2003; Yanos *et al.*, 2007). Simply put, structure refers to patterned social arrangements, in the form of institutions and power relations. Agency refers to the capacity of an individual to aspire, make choices and determine the direction of their life. The relationship between structure and agency is dialectic. Patterned social arrangements shape individual's actions and identities to varying degrees, while individual's actions, individually and collectively, can change social arrangement to differing extents.

The dominant recovery discourse underplays social factors and emphasises the agency side of recovery, i.e. promoting empowerment with an emphasis on a hopeful life, as advocated by the proponents of the Recovery Movement (e.g. Anthony, 1993, cited in DoH, 2009). It fails however to address the structural forces and social inequalities leading to ill health in the first place. These are factors that constrain and facilitate the development and exercise of agency during the recovery process. Such inequalities manifest themselves in a variety of forms, for example, class relations, gender, ethnicity, psychiatric power, ableism and sanism (Weisser *et al.*, 2011). Ableism and sanism are ideologies and practices that assume 'normativity' against a divisive notion of abled body/mind (Campbell, 2009) as well as madness and irrationality (Chamberlain, 1978; Perlin, 2000; Morrow and Weisser, 2012). Perlin (1999) referred to 'sanism' as an irrational prejudice against people labelled as 'mentally ill'. 'Sanism' as a systematic form of oppression is often likened to racism and sexism. It is a structural inequality for its 'valuing of rational thinking and socially acceptable forms of behavior, and the subsequent ostracisation and/or punishment of people who do not or cannot conform' (Morrow and Weisser, 2012: 31). Thus analysis on sanism goes beyond a focus on stigmatising practices and attitudes at social interactional level. It looks at what social structure breed and sanction such stigma (Poole *et al.*, 2012). Sanism, ableism and other inequalities can limit an individual's life chances and capacity to exercise agency in making life decisions. Therefore, to take agency seriously, we need to look at what structural changes are necessary within and beyond mental health services (Hopper, 2007; Pilgrim, 2008). To put structure into the recovery approach is to turn what people recover from into an empirical enquiry.

In this study I draw on the Capabilities Approach as a heuristic framework (Sen, 1999; Nussbaum, 2000; Jackson, 2005; Sayer, 2012) to empirically inquire into what recovery is by exploring the interplay of structure and agency. The Capabilities Approach was devised by Amartya Sen for development studies to evaluate a country's development in terms of well-being and quality of life instead of gross economic gain. Later it was adapted to studies in 'developed' countries for policy development and evaluations in areas such as education, health, disability and employment (e.g. Walker, 2006; Saleeby, 2007;

Ruger, 2009; Orton, 2011; Lewis, 2012). It has been taken up in mental health studies by a variety of authors concerned with exploring the importance of social context in recovery as well as agency development (Hopper, 2007; Ware *et al.*, 2008; Davidson *et al.*, 2011; Barrow *et al.*, 2014). The Capabilities Approach understands capabilities as the substantive freedom an individual has rather than the ability they possess. The process of exercising choice is one dimension of substantive freedom. But for such freedom to be substantive it is necessary to consider the opportunities available to an individual. The Capabilities Approach also identifies how an individual is able to convert ability and resources into forms of doing and being that are valued by them (Robeyns, 2005). Such conversion factors could be the environments, institutions, social policies, and the welfare regime individuals live in (Robeyns, 2005; Hopper, 2007; Orton, 2011). In other words, conversion factors are the facilitators or the structural barriers that enable or disable an individual from achieving a valued way of living.

Used as an evaluation tool, the Capabilities Approach is not concerned with what an individual eventually chooses to do. Rather, it focuses on whether an individual has the life chances or 'exercisable opportunities' (Daniels, 2010) to live the life they want. Instead of using one specific benchmark as the outcome of progress, i.e. recovery in this study, the Capabilities Approach looks at the multi-dimensional nature of an individual's quality of life. To empirically address the questions 'What is recovery?' a service user's capabilities set can be seen as the evaluative space that shows what capabilities have increased and what capabilities have decreased along the recovery process. This formulation not only addresses Pilgrim's third meaning of recovery. It also has the potential to transcend the debate as to whether the social model of disability is applicable to mental ill health (Wallcraft and Hopper, 2015).

Adaptive preference is another key concept in the Capabilities Approach, which helps to address the interplay of structure and agency by not taking what recovery is at face value (Sen, 1984; Nussbaum, 2000; Khader, 2011). Adaptive preference refers to an individual's perception of the scope of life choices and preferences in life decision-making, both of which can be shaped and restricted by the disadvantages that they face. This resonates with the idea of the temporal process of structural conditioning in exploring the way structure shapes individual actions (S.J. Williams, 2003). In the mental health context, Wallcraft (2011) has shown that in studies of quality of life measures, people diagnosed with severe mental illness, such as schizophrenia, tend to underrate decreases in their quality of life compared with researchers using 'objective' quality of life measures. This underrating could be a result of service users adapting their aspirations because of their experiences being invalidated and excluded.

Thus, the concept of adaptive preference prompts a look beyond the face value of service users' answers to the question 'What is recovery?' If hope is an important element in journeying to recovery then an examination of the process of how individuals form their hopes or preferences is important in tracking how their valued 'doing and being' changes over time. This focuses attention on the symptoms, impairments, or social invalidations that arise from structural inequalities and become the barriers that result in the adaptation of preferences in life.

Whose recovery?

One way to turn the question 'What do people recover from?' into an empirical enquiry is to ask 'Whose recovery is it?' (Social Perspectives Network, 2007). The Social Perspectives Network's report shows how the recovery approach has both addressed and failed to address, issues of diversity such as gender, sexuality and ethnicity. Challenges in different areas of life include and go beyond mental health discrimination. Structural constraints for different groups of people are constituted of barriers arising from a range of power inequalities. The dominant recovery discourse in mental health policies fails to address the diversity of lives that people want to live. People who face, or are marginalised by, different inequalities have different answers to the question 'What is recovery?' These answers have implications for identifying the structural barriers that need to be removed to achieve the capabilities necessary for meaningful recovery. For this reason, this book explores what recovery entails for Chinese mental health service users in the UK as a case study that identifies the structural barriers they face in their recovery journeys.

There are three main reasons for choosing to study Chinese mental health service users living in the UK. First and foremost, as a Chinese woman from Hong Kong who lived in the UK for 7 years and has been a mental health service user in Hong Kong and the UK, my personal history drew me to this topic. While Chinese people form the majority in Hong Kong and are a minority in the UK, I realised that there are common experiences shared by service users in both places due to the dominance of Western bio-medical psychiatry in both societies. I find resonance in some of the critiques of psychiatric power raised by the service user movement, but I am equally aware that Chinese people's experiences differ from other service users in the UK and this is a relatively unexplored topic. What Chinese people need to 'recover from' could be shaped by their positioning as an ethnic minority in the UK and their quality of life, and their envisioning of what constitutes the good life could be restricted as a result. My awareness of the issues that service users and Chinese people may encounter in the UK means that I am well positioned to undertake my chosen case study and draw on my service user experiences in the production of knowledge. My linguistic ability and cross-cultural experiences as a service user enabled me to communicate, understand and relate to other Chinese mental health service users as an insider.

Second, not only are Chinese people invisible in the UK service user movement, they remain marginal in academic studies including those on mental health. This is despite the fact that Chinese people in the UK are a visible community in terms of their skin colour, their cuisine and the Chinatowns that have been established in major UK cities since large-scale immigration in the 1960s. Chinese community has settled in the UK for more than 150 years. In 2011 the size of the UK Chinese population was approximately 400,000 forming 0.7 of the total population, an increase from an estimate of 250,000 in the 2001 Census.

Invisibility could be due to Chinese people living in UK often being portrayed as a homogenous group who live independently and can cope for themselves. Chinese people have migrated from diverse place of origins, including the People Republic of China (the mainland China), Hong Kong, Taiwan, Malaysia, Vietnam etc. Chinese ethnic communities are often regarded as hard to reach, self-contained and performing well on health indicators in the West. Compared to other ethnic minority groups, racialised assumptions about Chinese communities being a compliant, hardworking 'model minority' persist in the UK and North America (Archer and Francis, 2005; Kwok, 2013). The relatively low profile of the Chinese in the mainstream UK mental health literature may also be due to this group being seen as non-problematic. In contrast with Black service users who are overrepresented in hospital admissions and whose position has led to inquiries into institutional racism in the mental health services (Care Quality Commission, 2010), Chinese people are under-represented in the mental health services (Wong and Cochrane, 1989; Li, 1991; Yeung *et al.*, 2012). Such a comparatively low utilisation rate is also found in America. This raises questions as to whether this under-representation is a result of a lower prevalence of mental ill health in Chinese communities, different cultural conceptualization of mental illness, stigma, different help-seeking behavior or a result of institutional barriers that prevent Chinese people accessing services (Kwok, 2013; Rochelle and Shardlow, 2014).

This invisibility also raises questions of whether and how the experience of Chinese people differs from other ethnic minority groups in using mental health services. In the UK, studies on different ethnic groups have different focuses, which reflect the differential treatment they receive: the coercive treatment received by African-Caribbean communities, their high rate of receiving schizophrenia diagnoses and its relation to the British post-slavery legacy (e.g. Fernando, 2002); the 'somatisation thesis' and Asian women (Goldberg *et al.*, 1997) or its critics questioning whether such a thesis is a stereotypical generalisation and reflection of the problematic of Western psychiatry mind–body dichotomy (Watters, 1996); the over-representation of Irish people in the psychiatric population, the higher psychiatric admission rate of Irish people than ethnic minority groups and the material and cultural factors contributing to the vulnerability of Irish people to mental ill health (Cochrane and Bal, 1989; Jones, 1997). Therefore, in terms of causation of mental ill health or the reaction from Western psychiatry, the working out of race inequalities in relation to Chinese communities could be different from other minority ethnic groups.

This is further supported by studies on inter-ethnic differences in (mental) health (e.g. Nazroo, 1997, 1998, 2003). Based on the Fourth National Survey of Ethnic Minorities, Nazroo demonstrated that ethnic differences and inequalities in health are highly related to socio-economic differentials, rather than genetic or cultural difference (Nazroo, 1998). This is manifested in the socio-economic patterns within ethnic groups, the socio-economic patterning of health across ethnic groups, how socio-economic conditions across the life course can influence current health, as well as the impact of racial harassment and discrimination on health and the resulting socio-economic exclusion (Nazroo, 2003). This points to the intersection of class and ethnicity, i.e. that socio-economic disadvantages and deprivation inter-relate closely racialised hierarchies of exclusion, spanning across the life cycle (Salway *et al.*, 2010). Some questions can be raised about Chinese communities if this class-ethnicity intersection is applied to understand the health status of Chinese communities. If the overall Chinese health indicators are better than other ethnic groups based on the survey on self-reported health (Sproston and Mindell, 2006), to what extent is this due to 'cultural differences' between the general Chinese population and other ethnic groups? Or how far does it mask significant socio-economic differences between ethnic groups as well as the differentiated patterns of health within Chinese communities?

While race equality is mentioned in mental health policy documents (DoH, 2009), there is a persistent marginalisation of race in welfare provision (Craig and Walker, 2012). Despite employing community development workers for different communities under the Delivering Race Equality programme (DoH, 2005), the marginalisation of these workers in service structures has rendered sustainable changes difficult. The invisibility of Chinese people raises the question of whether policy makers and services are equipped to meet the diverse and differentiated needs of Chinese mental health service users adequately. What recovery entails for Chinese people in the UK and what capabilities development is needed in contrast to majority and other ethnic minority groups requires empirical exploration. How racism works and intersects with other inequalities as a barrier and impacts on the recovery process of the Chinese mental health service users also needs examination.

The third reason for selecting Chinese people in the UK as a case study is to use the data generated to develop an alternative framework, which can address ethnic inequalities, diversity and recovery. The invisibility of Chinese communities as well as the racialised assumption about this group, reflect the problematic nature of a culturalist approach in understanding Chinese people's diverse needs (Chau, 2008; Chau *et al.*, 2012). Diversity within the Chinese communities was glossed over and a homogenous health behaviour and health belief based on 'traditional' Chinese culture has been assumed. Recognising heterogeneity in Chinese communities is important to the exploration of their diverse needs in terms of generational experiences of migration, languages, country of origins, class, gender and age. It is also central to an exploration of how conflicts and divisions within Chinese communities become factors leading to the distress and ill health that service users need to recover from. A culturalist approach can also lead to a stereotypical view of what Chinese mental health service users want for their recovery journey. Public discourse and the government's stance in treating paid work as the ultimate criteria of social inclusion restricts the capabilities development of both majority and minority service users (Powell, 2000). A culturalist approach can also be capabilities limiting if it pigeonholes what Chinese people can achieve, what life they aspire to and how they can pursue it. In addition, a culturalist approach masks the role of material inequalities in constituting the life chances of minority groups (Ratcliff, 2012; Viruell-Fuentes *et al.*, 2012). Thus a culturalist approach is limited to investigating what Chinese people need to recover from.

The Capabilities Approach accommodates diversity in its focus on an individual's capabilities set instead of what a person ultimately chooses to do. It does not concern with what ways of life one lives to be counted as 'socially included'. Its focus is on an individual's capabilities set instead of what a person ultimately chooses to do. In this study I link Intersectionality Analysis to the Capabilities Approach to increase the analytical power required to tease out what structural barriers hinder the capability development of an individual's recovery process. Intersectionality Analysis originated in the United State's third wave feminist movement, which criticised second wave feminism for its failure to recognise women's diversity in fighting for women's rights. This resulted in White women's experiences being mistakenly asserted as the norm and as a result women's rights advocacy was unable to ground the claims based on the experience of Black women. Intersectionality Analysis purports that 'race', as well as oppressions based on gender and class do not work separately from each other. Instead, they mutually shape social structure, individual experience, and embodied identity (Collins, 1998, Crenshaw, 1991; McCall, 2005; Walby, 2007). More recently notions of intersectionality have been applied to policy making in order to address multiple strands of equality (Parken and Young, 2008; Hankivsky and Cormier, 2011; Viruell-Fuentes *et al.*, 2012).

Looking at how class, gender, ethnicity and other power relations intersect and shape the recovery process of Chinese mental health service users in the UK can increase understandings of the different ways structural barriers and facilitators impact on the capabilities development of this group to live a meaningful life. Individuals are not just service users. Everyone lives in a matrix of social roles, embodying different identities and facing different inequalities in everyday life as well as achieving personhood. Axes of power relations foreground and limit the exercisable opportunities available to different groups of service users and also shape their life choice preferences. Contrary to a quantitative social determinant approach to mental health, Intersectionality Analysis makes visible the varied and complex ways different axes of oppression work, and explores the interplay of structure and agency, which is at the heart of a structural approach to recovery.

Central inquiries and method

This book thus asks Chinese service users in the UK what they are recovering from and where they are travelling to. Three questions steer the direction of this study.

Question 1: What are the Chinese mental health service users in this study recovering from and what do they recover into?

This question demarcates the empirical focus of the study. First, it looks into the processes and experiences leading to the deterioration of mental well-being of service users and the distress they experience. Second, it studies 'recovery' as capabilities development: what were the qualities of life and life chances service users had before their mental health crisis? How did their capabilities change over the recovery journey? These questions shed light on the social context and life stages in which the events leading to mental ill health happened, as well as, the situations in which service users strive to recover. They also enable the exploration of the recovery themes of Chinese service users, which may vary because of the different ways structural forces constitute the social locations individuals recover from and in.

Question 2: What hinders and facilitates the recovery process, and in particular how do class, gender, ethnicity and other structural influences intersect to shape outcomes?

This question explores what helped or deterred Chinese service users in the UK from developing capabilities on several levels. This study analyses what facilitates or hinders the regaining of mental well-being capability as well as the development of the capabilities lost as a result of mental distress and ill health. It also analyses the development of lost capabilities that lead to mental ill health in the first place as well as that of further capabilities that could be inhibited by the discrimination experienced because of an individual's mental health history. Psychiatric systems and other social services will be under scrutiny. Other institutions such as the labour market, workplace, family and educational settings are also considered to track the ways they shape the recovery.

Attention will be given to service users' decision-making processes, i.e. what choices were presented to them, how they perceive their opportunities and why they made certain choices. Through this analysis at the institutional level, the way in which class, gender, ethnicity, sanism, psychiatric power and other inequalities intersect to shape quality of life and life chances will also be examined. The way identities impinge on service user's decision-making and how they make sense of social locations and negotiate within a matrix of power relations will also be explored.

Question 3: What are service users' assessments of their recovery journeys so far, in terms of the extent to which they consider themselves recovered and their hopes for the future?

This question asks individuals for their reflections on their recovery journey over time. It is concerned with what recovery means to Chinese service users living in the UK: how they experience hope; the divergence and commonality in their worldviews; and how their hopes about recovery and their worldviews have changed over time. These areas are expected to shed light on the adaptive preferences of individuals as they have emerged from their experiences of mental ill health and during the recovery journey. The way in which class, gender, ethnicity, psychiatric power, sanism and other inequalities have shaped their perceptions and outlooks on life will also be a focus.

The aim to look at the recovery process and lived experience with a structure and agency analysis requires a research method that allows narratives to unfold and generates data about the impact of structuring forces on individual perceptions and actions. The issue of recovery from what to where, together with a focus on capabilities before ill health necessitates that the data collected should have a wider time frame than an 'illness narrative' approach with a focus on ill health (Kleinman, 1988; Hydén, 1997). For these reasons a biographical method is used, echoing the call from C. Wright Mills for a sociological imagination that 'deals with problems of biography, of history, and of their intersections within social structures' (2000: 143).

Biographical method (or 'life story' or 'life history', which are used interchangeably in this book) allows for the collection of data that demonstrates the interaction of biography and social structure. As Bertaux put it, it is about 'what people have done, where and when, with whom, with which context, with which results. They are also about what has been done to those people, and how they reacted' (2003: 39–40).

To capture the variety of Chinese service users experiences in the UK, as well as exploring how different structural factors impact on capabilities development along their recovery journeys, purposive sampling was employed to recruit Chinese service users with diverse backgrounds in terms of received diagnoses, gender, place of birth and class status (Oliver, 2006). I aimed to ensure heterogeneity among the sample to explore how different social locations had shaped their recovery journeys. As this study aimed to explore markers in developing a structural approach to recovery and to understand how various structural factors work, a sample of Chinese service users with pluralities of experiences of mental health problems and social backgrounds were recruited to allow for detailed analysis. To ensure plurality, there were only two recruitment criteria. These were self-identification as Chinese and having received a psychiatric diagnosis. The term 'having received a diagnosis' was used to take into account individuals who might not identify themselves as being mental health patients or service users. I wanted to include people who rejected their diagnosis or the treatments they had been prescribed in order to explore and understand their position. One innovation in the research design is that I decided to include myself as one of the participants. Reflections on the reason behind this decision, ethical considerations, as well as challenges arisen and strategies taken in the fieldwork will be elaborated in the methodological epilogue. Altogether there were 22 service users (including myself) being recruited and interviewed between 2009 and 2010. They were mainly recruited through Chinese community centres in Birmingham, London and Manchester. Among the participants, there were sojourners coming to study in recent years and second generation who were born in the UK. Yet, the majority of participants reflected the more vulnerable population in the Chinese communities who sought help from community centres because of their lack of English speaking skills and being the first-generation migrants experiencing isolation. (See the Appendix for a background of the participants under pseudonyms and Chapter 3 for the general demographic information of this group).

I prepared an interview topic guide for the in-depth interview, covering areas of life relevant to the recovery journeys of the participants. General information about the participants were captured during each interview, for example, whether they were British born or migrants, the countries they had lived in before migrating to the UK, age, work history, marital status, status of residency in the UK, diagnosis received and living arrangements. The interview strategy involved two parts. The first part aimed to enable participants to recount their stories by posing open questions. The second part aimed to focus on exploring how different power inequalities had shaped the recovery journey through asking more focused questions based on the social locations of the participants.

I started each interview with the opening 'I would like to understand your recovery journey. Can you tell me about it?' to give participants space to tell their stories. Asking them to recount stories with this open question was intended as an invitation to them to reminisce and provide a picture of their life history. Then I asked about what happened before, during and after the mental health incidents they mentioned, in order to contextualise the mental health problems in their life history as well as understand how they exercised agency or if their agency had been compromised. Attention was paid to narratives about decision-making processes to solicit the ways in which they made sense of mental health incidents, the resources and social networks they had, the strategies they employed, the barriers they encountered and the perceived choices and possibilities they had. Through this strategy, I hoped to get a sense of the following from the participants:

1   What did they recover from in terms of distress, symptoms, as well as the social determinants triggering their mental health problem?
2   What did they recover into, i.e. their current being and doing, and their current livelihood?
3   What would they want to do/be now and in the future? How had their life goals changed over the years?
4   What were the changes in their capabilities and life chances across their life history as a result of their mental health problem and inequalities related to class, gender, ethnicity, age and disability?

I wanted the data generated in each of these areas to build up a picture of what and how capabilities had changed along the recovery journey and life history, as well as the social locations of the participants. Information about social locations would then help me to carry out the second part of the interview, which would explore further how different power inequalities had shaped the facilitators or barriers to capability development. This further exploration could be carried out in the same interview or in a follow-up interview following the transcription and analysis of the first interview. This second part of the interview also allowed me to validate my interpretation, e.g. the social locations of the participants as well as the significance of different factors on the participants' recovery journey, by asking more focused questions.

Apart from using life history interviews as the primary data collection method, other methods were employed to enrich my understanding of the social context the participants lived in. Observation was carried out whenever possible. This involved attending activities held for the service users by Chinese community centres, accompanying and assisting service users in local consultation events as an interpreter, or visiting their homes if I was invited and if I judged it appropriate. These observations helped me to become familiar with the lives of participants at the time of the interviews.

A documentary search helped me to contextualise and embed the participants' recovery journeys and biographies in macro social history and structure. Ensuring the embeddedness of the biography can help illustrate the workings of social mechanisms (Chamberlayne *et al.*, 2000). The search included social histories of Chinese communities in the UK, covering migration history, social mobility structures, changes in the climate of racial discrimination and immigration policies as well as the social history of the countries they migrated too. All were important to embedding the biographies of the participants in order to generate a rounded analysis.

Recovery from what to where?

In this book recovery is viewed as a process, a standpoint advocated by service users in the recovery movement. Service user literature stresses recovery as a non-linear process that is unique to each individual (Ridgway, 2001; Davidson *et al.*, 2005). As Deegan describes recovery, 'at times our course is erratic and we falter, slide back, re-group and start again' (1988: 15). Despite setbacks, or relapses, in this process, there is a sense of 'turning to' a better state away from withdrawal, despair and patienthood (Ridgway, 2001; Wallcraft, 2001). Turning to, suggests human agency as users actively pursue their recovery journey and personal growth. 'Hope' is emphasised in the recovery literature in relation to the restoration and development of users' agency against the dampening of the human spirit, which can result from mental ill health, invalidation and the denial of a better life associated with patienthood. In sum the recovery process is an ongoing journey (Ridgway, 2001) – with a sense of movement from a state of restrictive patienthood to meaningful personhood, yet the pace and desired direction of travel is determined by the user. Facilitating recovery thus means facilitating the agency development of service users to drive their own recovery journeys. To recover means moving from what restricts them as they pursue a life they value.

Metaphors used in the Tidal model stimulate our imagination in understanding the interplay of agency and structure that shape the travelling of a recovery journey (Barker and Buchanan-Barker, 2005). The Tidal model emphasises personhood, i.e. an understanding of madness or mental illness as part of the process of being human. It uses 'flowing water', 'ocean' and 'seafaring' as metaphors to describe its existential view of human experience and everyday life. Although the Tidal model was conceptualised in the Western world, this use of water and waves as metaphors is not only found in English usage. It is also found in Eastern philosophies such as Buddhism and Taoism (Lai, 1979). While the ebbs and flows of one's life signal the non-linear nature of the recovery journey, the metaphors used in the Tidal model are also useful to demarcate the various stages experienced in a recovery voyage. 'Drowning' is when a person experiences acute distress. The prelude to drowning is 'things falling apart', as if a ship has begun to lose its ability to navigate and stay afloat on the ocean of experiences. The comparison of the robustness of a ship to an individual's well-being can avoid the contested dichotomies between body and mind, and physical and mental health. Mental health care, as an ideal, is likened to a 'safe haven' that prepares an individual to return to the oceans of experience after a shipwreck (Barker and Buchanan-Barker, 2005: 21–23). Agency can be understood as the service user taking control of the helm and reading the bearings and assessing the weather, wind directions and current flow in order to steer in their chosen direction of travel.

The role of social forces goes beyond individual attributed characteristics or immediate social contexts as implicated in the individualistic bio-psycho-social model. It concerns the multidimensional structural forces that impinge on the direction of the recovery journey. The interplay of structural forces results in the variations of recovery journeys. To understand what exactly users recover from is to understand what and how the strong waves or ocean's currents result in shipwreck and adverse conditions from which an individual can re-embark on their life journey. Their experiences in a safe haven also impact on the extent to which service users are able to exercise agency and take the helm in their life voyage. What, then, are the social forces shaping the Chinese service users' recovery journeys?

Possible social forces impinging on Chinese service users' recovery journeys

The following literature review provides a glimpse of the social forces known, and what is yet to be explored, in relation to 1) what contributes to the distress and mental ill health of Chinese people; 2) their experiences of accessing (mental) health services; and 3) what facilitates or hinders their recovery journeys in rebuilding their lives. In reviewing the literature, I will also identify gaps in these researches and discuss how they relate to this study.

What contributes to the distress and mental ill health of Chinese people in the UK

Huang and Spurgeon (2006) and Lane *et al.* (2010) explicitly addressed the issue of mental ill health and contributive social factors leading to mental ill health. Huang and Spurgeon (2006) looked at sources of psychological distress for Chinese migrants in Birmingham. Language and communication problems were identified as a source of distress when individuals had to deal with legal and formal procedures concerning matters such as employment. Workers in the Chinese catering industry saw English proficiency as irrelevant to their well-being but felt isolated from their Chinese friends because of the scattered geographical locations of Chinese restaurants in the UK. Aging and marital breakdown were also identified as sources of distress. Those who befriended British people, experienced a cultural gap with their friends, and at the same time felt distanced from the support of Chinese people. Interestingly, the respondents in this study described this tension and isolation as necessary to their personal struggle to succeed professionally in the UK. At the same time the majority of them reported racial discrimination. However the correlation between discrimination and poor mental health was not found to be statistically significant. This, as the authors note, contrasts with the findings of Karlsen and Nazroo (2002) who reported a strong relationship between poor health and perceptions of racial discrimination.

This discrepancy raises interesting questions about how Chinese people perceived and experienced discrimination. For example, while unfair treatment at work was clearly identified, it was often seen as a personal problem resulting from a lack of having a strong enough competitive spirit, rather than a disadvantage resulting from the dominance of White normality or institutional racism. In what ways does such personalisation and internalisation help legitimise the structural racism and become a source of stress for the Chinese people? A study by Adamson *et al.* (2009) found that Chinese people identified overt discrimination such as verbal abuse and attacks more readily than the disadvantages they experienced in the workplace. Victims of racial attacks reported resulting psychological distress and mental health problems. Distrust of the police as a source of help and protection was also reported. Yet, whether it is covert or overt racial discrimination, the psychological impact can be profound. Tong et al (2014) found that Chinese people are the minority suffering from the highest level of 'race' hate crime.

In terms of employment, adverse work conditions, precarious employment and immigration status have been linked to mental ill health in the literature. These factors reflected structural forces such as changing economic conditions and its impact on the anti-immigration climate and subsequent tightening of immigration controls. Exploitation in terms of low pay has been found to negatively impact on the psychological well-being of migrants (Pharoah and Lau, 2009). Wu *et al.* (2010) demonstrated how these factors are worsening because of economic recession. They found employers were manipulating the immigration system to exploit the workers, through unfair punishment and coercion. For example, abusing the desperation of work permit holders for whom application for permanent residency is contingent on having continuous employment in the UK. Deterioration of mental health and feelings of hopelessness were found to be commonly experienced in relation to poor working conditions. Employer abuse towards work permit holders was rife, with one victim being hospitalised with a mental health problem.

In terms of social networks, the 'double social exclusion' highlighted by Chau and Yu (2001) dispelled the myth that Chinese people can 'take care of themselves' because they are a close-knit community. Social exclusion is doubled when individuals experience separation from British people as well as other Chinese people. To participate in the UK economy Chinese catering businesses are geographically spread to maximise profits through minimising competition. This physical distance is coupled with social distance for employees as these small businesses are also tight family units. This evidence counters culturalist assumptions about the behaviour of Chinese people. It shows that notwithstanding self-identification as Chinese and shared customs or cultural activities, it is material conditions that prevent some Chinese workers from forming supportive networks.

There are two studies that have looked at Chinese women in the UK and discussed the role of gender in relation to well-being, using an intersectionality lens (implicitly and explicitly) for analysis (Lee *et al.*, 2002; Lane *et al.*, 2010). Lee *et al.* (2002) looked at the way women negotiate their gendered and racialised migration trajectories with different cultural and economic capitals. Women who come to the UK as the brides of Chinese or White British men were shown to possess less cultural and economic capital than women who came to the UK with their family or as independent migrants. Brides were more vulnerable to isolation and dependence on their spouses and stressed by the heavy domestic demands made on them as well as their strained relationships with their in-laws. This study analysed the way structural inequalities shaped the acculturation experiences of woman migrants between the 1960s and 1970s and traced how this subsequently contributed to the predicaments this group experienced in their old age. Their marginality in the labour market at a time of acute gendered and ethnic division of labour in the UK, their unpaid labour in family businesses, their lack of English language skills and their distance from children who did not identify with Chinese cultures meant that they did not have the financial security of a retirement pension to live on and they suffered from isolation in their old age. These women were also at risk of having poor mental health.

Lee *et al.* (2002) provide a background for devising a way of exploring the social forces that constitute what Chinese service users recover from. This approach challenges the culturalist assumption made about Chinese communities in the UK. It privileges social determinants over life style in discussing the impact of social factors on mental health (Marmot *et al.*, 2010). It draws on the usefulness of using an intersectionality lens in illustrating the ways multidimensional structural inequalities forces intersect to contribute to distress. Lane *et al.* (2010) illustrate how ethnicity as structure, compounded with gender relations, impact on mental health. Karlsen and Nazroo (2002) used quantitative measures to show that it was ethnicity as structure in terms of racialisation and class experience, rather than ethnicity as identity, that was strongly associated with health for ethnic minorities in the UK.

Understanding ethnicity as structure puts emphasis on the interplay of structural factors in constituting socio-economic deprivation and its consequence on health for ethnic minorities. As Salway *et al.* (2010) argue in response to the Marmot review (2010), this offers a better explanation of the impact of social factors on health for ethnic minorities than looking at the effect of social determinants one by one. The socio-economic deprivation that ethnic minorities in the UK face inter-relates with exclusion and discrimination resulting from racialised hierarchies. Lane *et al.* (2010) have enriched understandings of the socio-economic deprivation faced by ethnic minority women through looking at how the gendered division of labour intersects with the ethnic structure in a globalised world.

The experience of Chinese people accessing mental health services

Literature concerning Chinese peoples' access to mental health services addresses their help-seeking behaviours, health beliefs, social networks, the barriers encountered in accessing health services, cultural (in)sensitivity, multicultural services and medical pluralism. Yeung *et al.* (2012) argue that the relatively low rate of use of mental health services in primary care by Chinese people compared to other ethnic groups, is a matter of the under-utilisation of community level services rather than a lack of need for services. While the hospital admission rates of Chinese mental health service users were found to be lower than average, compulsory admissions (67 per cent) were higher than average (47 per cent). This means that, compared to the national average, Chinese service users were more likely to come into contact with mental health services when they were in crisis, resulting in their hospitalisation through Accident and Emergency Units of General Hospitals (Care Quality Commission, 2010; cited in Yeung *et al.*, 2012: 2). The factors that have been identified in a range of studies as reasons for the under utilisation of health services include language barriers, tendencies not to identify psychological distress or somatic symptoms in terms of mental illness and fear of stigma. (e.g. Li and Logan, 1999; Green *et al.*, 2002; Tran *et al.*, 2008).

Communication barriers, as Green *et al.* (2002) indicated in their study, are linguistic as well as conceptual in nature and result in difficulties engaging in meaningful dialogue with practitioners to explain psychological distress. They called for improvements in the quality and quantity of interpretation and advocacy services that can act as 'cultural brokers' (p. 220). Li and Logan (1999) and

Tran *et al.* (2008) argue for the provision of mental health promotion materials in Chinese languages, explaining what psychiatric disorders are and information about mental health services in Chinese languages. Tran *et al.* (2008) also called for more mental health professionals with Chinese-speaking abilities to be made available across different constituencies.

Other studies have looked at the health beliefs and explanatory models used by Chinese people in the UK and discussed their relation to help-seeking behaviours. They argue against a static view of health beliefs that assume Chinese people prefer to use or believe in Traditional Chinese medicine and its concepts based on the philosophy of Confucianism and Taoism (Yip, 2005). Traditional Chinese medicine understands health and well-being as a balance and harmony between yin and yang, a good flow of chi (energy) and advocates the restraint of emotions.

Green *et al.* (2006) showed that Chinese migrants draw upon both Western and Traditional Chinese medicine and their explanatory models, in the UK and their homelands. The ways they used these two models varied. This fluid use was seen as maximising their health resources. The fluid, mixed use of explanatory models by Chinese migrants was shaped by their exposure in China to both medical models. This reflected a long history in which Chinese societies have been exposed to foreign medical practices (Yu, 2006). The availability of Traditional Chinese medicine practitioners and the means to pay for Chinese medicine in the UK or fly back to their country of origin for treatments were important factors in the use of Chinese medicine (Lai Yin Association, 1999).

Studies have also suggested that a multicultural approach at institutional and practitioner levels is required to address the health needs of the Chinese in the UK. Green *et al.* (2006) argue for medical pluralism to make Chinese medicine an available treatment of option in mainstream public health services, while Chau *et al.* (2011) argue for the importance of recognising the diverse health needs within Chinese communities and suggested analytical tools that practitioners could employ to find out about the health needs and beliefs of individuals (e.g. culturagram). Yeung *et al.* (2012) explored the role of social networks in help-seeking and found that family members may not be involved in every stage of the help-seeking pathway. This is an important focus in understanding how relations enable or constrain service users in seeking help from statutory health services and other sources. All these studies suggest the need for practitioners to proactively understand the diverse needs of this marginalised group, especially when Chinese people felt that their voices would not be listened to regarding their concerns and dissatisfaction with services (Yeung *et al.*, 2015).

In sum, this literature is concerned with the (lack of) multicultural services in the UK and proposes improvements aimed at increasing practitioners' understandings of the needs of Chinese people by improving their cultural competencies and sensitivity. As dominant White culture and the minority cultures do not meet on equal terms (Ahmad and Atkin, 1996), what makes one medical model dominant and others 'alternative' and what diagnosis classification is adopted are historical socio-political processes involving the state and professional power. In this context medical pluralism is rightly advocated.

Yet, one limitation of this literature is that it frames the nature of inequalities experienced by Chinese people using services as being due to ethnic inequality. Scant attention has been paid to the problematic care and control role psychiatry has through its medicalisation of human suffering and its exercise of state sanctioned coercion (Fernando, 2002). A large gap in the UK literature relates to the ways medicalisation enables or hinders Chinese users' achievement of meaningful recovery. The unequal power relation in psychiatry between service users and professionals is also related to the dominance of (Western) bio-medical understandings of human suffering. Medication is the predominant treatment available to mental health service users. When asked about its impact on their recovery some service users say they find it enabling, others find it disabling while some have a mixed experience of it (Southside Partnership/Fanon, 2008; Kalathil *et al.*, 2011a). While proposing that medical pluralism is one way to challenge the dominance of Western bio-medical model, what is lacking is a critique of the restricted view of normality Western and Chinese societies perpetuate by their use of the (Western and Chinese) bio-medical model.

To understand how the process of medicalisation shapes recovery journeys, it is important to delineate racism and the unequal power relations between service users and professionals and then explore the relation between the two. For example, Fernando (2006) argues that the unstated job description of professional staff to control people seen as deviant or dangerous can operate with racist assumptions in the diagnostic process, which is in turn embedded in psychiatric stigma. While this observation is usually used to explain the overrepresentation of Black African and Caribbean people in the UK mental health system, it should not be assumed that racism or an ethnocentric assumption of normalcy do not impact on the diagnoses received by Chinese service users. In addition, analytically separating the power relations and inequalities between service users and professionals (and the mental health services as a system) from other forms of power inequalities allows scope to investigate how other power dimensions in terms of, for example, gender, class, heterosexism and ageism, shape the medicalisation process and the direction of recovery journeys (Morrow and Wessier, 2012).

What facilitates or hinders service users' journeys in rebuilding their lives?

There is no literature on Chinese users in the UK that looks at recovery in a systematic way. To explore the possible social forces in this phase of recovery, I will review the literature that discusses recovery in relation to social inclusion, social integration and social recovery in general, as well as those that explicitly discuss social factors and recovery in the UK context.

The first literature comprises studies that aim to establish baselines for practitioners and services to facilitate social inclusion of service users. For example, three elements of the model were advocated in Repper and Perkins (2003). Facilitating personal adaptation is important so that service users can gain control over their mental health problems and their lives. Promoting access to valued social roles and material resources and creating hope-inspiring relationships is crucial. Power imbalances between users and professionals need to be addressed to achieve these.

Davidson *et al.* (2001) argue that social inclusion should mean 'to be let in' without being judged for adequacy and the three elements that set the foundation for this are friendship, being able to reciprocate in relationships and hope and affirmation. Borg and Davidson (2008) discussed what recovery means for everyday living. They concluded that service users envision desired everyday living through comparing what they called 'being normal', with variations of what exactly 'normal' means to them. Ware *et al.* (2007, 2008) argued for an understanding of social integration as quality of life, connectedness and citizenship. Indeed, enjoying the rights and citizenships that others have were advocated throughout this literature.

For Chinese people in the UK, establishing an understanding of citizenship for service users may entail more than the challenge of mental health discrimination. For new migrants, changing immigration policy means that the criteria to apply for permanent residency in the UK are constantly shifting. Their struggle for rights and entitlements in terms of citizenship thus also entails a dimension that is related to nationality.

Three studies go beyond generating baselines for inclusion and ask what social factors hinder or facilitate service users' achievement of a better life. Tew *et al.* (2012) review literature around 'connectedness', 'identities' and 'empowerments'. Three key messages emerge from this review, which are relevant to this book. First, exploring social factors that facilitate recovery requires tackling those that contribute to ill health in the first place. Second, tackling mental health discrimination and rebuilding a positive self and social identity are interlinked with racial discrimination, gender relations and identities. Third, discrimination and barriers service users encounter can worsen the distress and ill health they experience, as well as exacerbating the challenges they already have to deal with alongside their persisting mental health difficulties.

Some social factors as well as related practices to facilitate recovery highlighted by the authors are relevant too. Closely linked to 'empowerment' is the context of power relations. Individually, the strengths approach helps service users identify and mobilise their resources. For members of ethnic minorities this also means making positive use of their cultural resources (Jones *et al.*, 2007, cited in Tew *et al.*, 2012: 447), while individual budgets enable people to self-direct the supports they need to do this. To facilitate empowerment at a collective level, mutual or service user run services can provide more participatory and less hierarchical environments in which strategies learnt from experience can be shared.

In terms of identity, studies of ethnic minority communities indicate that discrimination due to race and mental illness co-exist, intensify each other and are experienced together. This means that recovery entails tackling both (Armour *et al.*, 2009; Scottish Recovery Network, 2008; Southside Partnership/Fanon, 2008; all cited in Tew *et al.*, 2012: 449). Gender identity can act in a paradoxical way. While service users may resort to gender identity to rebuild a life away from self-stigma, this strategy may reinforce the dominant gender stereotypes that contributed to their mental health difficulties in the first place (Emslie *et al.*, 2006, cited in Tew *et al.*, 2012: 449). Discrimination also operates at a structural level such as housing and employment (Corrigan *et al.*, 2004, cited in Tew *et al.*, 2012: 449).

As for ensuring 'connectedness' against social isolation, it is acknowledged that the quality of relationship matters. Participation in meaningful activities in communities, a sense of belonging in family and communities and being employed are usually seen as positive to recovery. However, it is worth noting that some service users find maintaining too much family connection stressful, especially when they need space to cope with mental health difficulties (Boydell *et al.*, 2002, cited in Tew *et al.*, 2012: 453). Tackling this requires service users to negotiate with family members for change and understanding. In addition, rather than seeing employment or participation in communities as ends in themselves, their positive or negative impact on recovery and well-being needs to be carefully researched. Tew *et al.* (2012), agreeing with Mezzina *et al.* (2006), argue that 'choices' of ways to participate for social inclusion is crucial so that service users can choose activities that are meaningful and helpful to them.

Two studies look at the experiences of Black men and Black and South Asian women in the UK respectively (Southside Partnership/Fanon, 2008; Kalathil *et al.*, 2011a). Both put inequalities at the heart of the discussion, attending to how service users attributed social disadvantages as the causes of their mental health difficulties and how they exacerbated the barriers to recovery. Southside Partnership/Fanon (2008) asked male African and African Caribbean service users living in the UK about the barriers to, and facilitators of, their recovery. Their findings resonate with much of the baseline literature reviewed earlier.

Although this study focussed on men, it did not explicitly discuss gender relation and identity in relation to recovery. Kalathil *et al.* (2011a) explicitly addressed gender as a social factor and so illustrated how gender and race discrimination within communities and wider society shape the experience of mental distress and the inequalities encountered when using mental health services. Gendered norms can impact on women's help-seeking behaviours. Some women were found to have internalised submissiveness and accepted being depressed as a normal state. While for others, the perceived image of women having strong emotions burdened them unnecessarily with notions of being resilient and therefore not asking for help. Thus oppression from gendered norms is what some women had to recover from, as they do not conform to societal expectations. The authors therefore argued for a 'transcultural approach to recovery' entailing 'understandings of distress as legitimate responses to life events, spiritual crises, "breakdown" due to trauma and stress and other cultural and personal explanations' (Kalathil et al. 2011a: 75). Creating safe spaces for service users to make sense, share and discuss these issues was identified as important to this work.

To sum up, the picture presented by the literatures reviewed in this chapter indicate the social conditions that contribute to distress and mental ill health, as well as those that pose challenges to achieving meaningful recovery cannot be tackled or rectified by an individualistic social approach that stresses developing users' social and coping skills. The social condition that Chinese people in the UK live in is one that has both a national and transnational dimension.

The above baselines and related social factors serve as useful pointers for this study to identify possible social relations, networks and institutions that constitute the social conditions that Chinese service users recover in. They serve as an entry point to analysing how structural forces shape these social relations, networks and institutions that subsequently become barriers or facilitators in recovery journeys. The social forces and inequalities that contribute to distress and mental ill health for Chinese service users in the first place need to be examined to see whether and how they develop strategies to deal with these causes, and whether they exacerbate the challenges service users encounter in their recovery. Chinese service users can experience mental health stigma and discrimination within Chinese communities and in mainstream society. Gender, class and ethnicity can interplay with mental health stigma and discrimination in constituting a notion of 'norms' linked to sanism and ableism, as well as social practices, services and policies that can be exclusionary. Strategies that Chinese service users employ to (re)develop a meaningful life might be related to their gendered and racialised identities.

Overview of the book

This book consists of seven chapters. Chapter 2 further discusses how the synthesis of the Capabilities Approach and Intersectionality Analysis, underpinned by a critical realist ontology, will guide the analysis of the Chinese people's recovery journey.

Chapters 3 to 6 focus on different phrases of the recovery journey. Chapter 3 introduces the participants in the context of the social history of Chinese communities in the UK. It portrays the events and predicaments giving rise to the deterioration of their mental well-being. The different axes of power inequalities that shaped the social locations of the participants and contributed to the diminishment of their mental well-being capability are analysed.

Chapter 4 sheds light on the myriad capabilities-enhancing or capabilities-debilitating ways participants navigated, stumbled along or were coerced into mental health care. Meanings will be attended to, so as to show how the participants grappled with the various parts of the psychiatric system and in what way the services helped or hindered recovery. Through discussing the pathologisation process and the discrepancy between the participants' own explanatory models and psychiatry's medicalisation framework, the intersection of power relations will also be illustrated. A close look is taken at how the participants experienced the psychiatric system and the ways psychiatric power and sanism begin to become structuring forces on their subsequent life journeys.

Chapter 5 explores the flow of the recovery journey begun after a crisis or an acute period of mental ill health. It explores the experience of participants in using the statutory and voluntary services to find out what helped and hindered their recovery process. Through looking at how participants rebuilt their lives in different areas, the intersection of structural factors, such as sanism and ableism, in the constitution of their new social locations is examined as are the different set of life chances that participants faced.

Chapter 6 reveals how participants adapt their recovery and life goals in response to their changed capabilities set. The ways in which participants use different identities in the face of the discriminations they experience are analysed. Hope, an important element in the recovery approach, is explored through the participants' lived experiences and articulations of hope.

Chapter 7 concludes with an overview of the way social conditions conducive or unfavorable to the recovery of Chinese service users. I will discuss policy and service implications concerning mental health services in general and Chinese service users in particular. Through this I argue for a social justice agenda to tackle social inequalities for meaningful recovery.

The book will end with a methodological epilogue reflecting on the fieldwork process in relation to the development of service user knowledge in Chinese communities. A reflexive account is given of how I used my experience as a service user who has lived in Hong Kong and the UK in my role as researcher. The issues of language, translations and ethical considerations taken will be discussed. Challenges encountered during the fieldwork will be reflected upon to discuss issues on building a collective capability of knowledge development for Chinese communities.

2   Exploring social inequalities with the Capabilities Approach and Intersectionality Analysis

Introduction

Before embarking on the journeys of the Chinese service users, this chapter elaborates on the choice of theoretical frameworks employed in this study of recovery, ethnic minorities and inequalities. A critical realist exploration is employed rather than traditional social causation or a constructivist model. This leads to the choice to use the Capabilities Approach and Intersectionality Analysis in this study. Whether and how the recovery journey entails the *development* or *diminishment* of service users' capabilities to achieve their valued 'doing' and 'being' will be analysed, using the Capabilities Approach. Intersectionality Analysis is used to address *what* hinders or facilitates recovery and *how* class, gender, ethnicity and other structural influences intersect to shape outcomes, i.e. the direction of the recovery journey travels and the capabilities individuals have. The last section of this chapter provides an account of how the synthesis of these two theories will be used to guide the exploration and understanding of the journeys of Chinese service users.

A critical realist exploration

While the aim of this study is to look at the social in recovery, it does not take a simplistic 'social causation' model underpinned by a traditional 'realist' framework that accepts 'medical naturalism' and does not consider psychiatric constructs as problematic (Pilgrim and Bentall, 1999; Rogers and Pilgrim, 2010). Critiques of medical naturalism do not just come from critical research about ethnic minorities and culture. Research based on service users' experiences in Anglo-Saxon countries and those researchers who hold a social constructionist view (e.g. Szasz, 1971) are also critical of Western psychiatry as a hegemonic system that shapes our understandings of mental health and madness and, in turn, how best to help people in distress.

Cross-cultural psychiatric research traces the medicalisation of madness and distress in different countries, e.g. how Western-specific ethnocentric diagnoses are universalised (e.g. Kleinman, 1977; Fernando, 2003). Western bio-medical psychiatry is not only hegemonic in respect to non-Western cultures or ethnic minorities in the West. Constructivists problematise medical naturalism that promotes a disease model of mental illness. Szasz (1961) argue that mental illness is a metaphor that is used to legitimise state control through the psychiatric professions and mental health laws. Medicalisation is a way to mask the problems of living. Autobiographies and narratives written by service users can be seen as protest literature against psychiatric hegemony (Hornstein, 2009). The problem with Szasz's position is that it concludes that people with distress and mental ill health should be left alone in society and so promotes moral and political nihilism; and thus is unable to offer praxis in dealing with suffering that is real or tackling social conditions that give rise to it (Sedgwick, 1982; Pilgrim, 2016). Another strand of constructivism links with post-structuralism and deconstruction (e.g. Parker *et al.*, 1997). Its concerns are to expose the production of psychiatric knowledge and its relation to power through a focus on discursive practice. However, the limitation of this emphasis on the role of discourse is that it implies only discourse is 'knowable' and rejects any claims about 'reality' (Pilgrim, 2013). Such a position offers limited insights to understandings of the social causes of psychological distress and mental ill health.

In the light of my criticisms of the simplistic social causation model and constructivism, this study employs critical realism to retain the strength of realism and constructivism (Bhaskar, 1989; Sayer, 1992; Archer, 2000; Rogers and Pilgrim, 2010; Pilgrim, 2015), which maintains a commitment to enquire into the 'real bodies and real selves, real lives and real worlds' (S.J. Williams, 1999: 813). The emphasis of critical realism in explaining phenomenon with material reality (structure) invites consideration of 'generative mechanisms' to unravel the social conditions individuals live in that lead to the deterioration of their mental health and shapes their recovery journeys (Higgs *et al.*, 2004). Generative or causal mechanisms are not analysed through the frequency of the occurrence of an event, or whether events happen in a particular sequence. Causal relationships lie not in events but in generative mechanisms that produce the events. While the systemworld is embedded in the lifeworld, they are not analytically conflated. The former concerns systems such as markets, bureaucracy and the law while the latter concerns lived experience and discourse. They are distinct because the former, as Sayer puts it, has a 'logic and momentum of its own which partly escapes the conscious mediation by actors' (1999: 319).

Thus a critical realist approach brings culture to this study of Chinese people in the UK. The notion of generative mechanisms allows the analysis of culture – 'social and cultural embedding of particular instances of systems and the cultural mediations of their effects' (Sayer, 1999: 321). A critical realist exploration also allows for the role of 'meaning' in analysis. In the context of this study, where the voices of Chinese service users and how they make sense of their recovery journeys are explored, the focus of standpoint theorisation is compatible with critical realist epistemology (Collins, 1998; Harding, 1998). Starting from the standpoint of service users (or ethnic minorities) does not necessarily lead to a deconstruction project that risks resulting in a nihilist consumerist notion of a pluralism of viewpoints; nor does it necessarily ignore the possibility of false consciousness or what the Capabilities Approach understands as 'adaptive preference'.

In developing an emancipatory conceptualisation of indigeneity, Kjosavik (2011) argues that a standpoint is 'not self-evident or obvious to someone by virtue of being merely a member of the subordinate social group; one has to struggle for it' (p. 120). 'To struggle for it' means that for standpoints to become useable knowledge, a participatory, reflexive, and often political, project is necessary for members of a group to collectively make sense of their experiences through challenging hegemonic ideologies and beliefs. The ability to reflect is a property of 'being human' and central to critical realism (Archer, 2000). This does not exclude people labelled as 'mad', as illustrated by the burgeoning mental health service user literature. Such a view asserts the role of agency in understanding of recovery journeys.

While this study privileges service user's perspectives to understand their lived experiences and the social conditions that shape their recovery journeys, a caution is noted here on the relation of social forces and mental ill health and distress. The multilevel generative mechanism (biological, psychological and social) in relation to mental health may not always be captured in personal accounts. The contingent and conjunctural causality of these plural generative mechanisms could lie outside the consciousness of the person. Thus what this study aims to achieve is a context-specific inquiry (Pilgrim, 2014). It is through understanding a localised social context that I attempt to explore pointers of *possible* social forces pertinent to the emergence of mental ill health and distress for this particular ethnic minority group.

To ground this study in a critical realist exploration, in order to understand the complex interplay of structure and agency, requires additional analytical frameworks to build an experiential understanding of recovery as an ongoing journey. To link lifeworld to systemworld, the Capabilities Approach and Intersectionality Analysis are used as theoretical frameworks. With the Capabilities Approach, a recovery journey as a move away from patienthood to personhood is understood as a development of capabilities. The Capabilities Approach is used as a heuristic framework to explore the social conditions for recovery for Chinese people in the UK. Intersectionality is used to explore the generative mechanisms leading to the expansion, diminishment or deprivation of one's capabilities.

Five reasons for using the Capabilities Approach

The Capabilities Approach, developed by Sen (1999) is a normative theory about what human development should be and how to access it. As opposed to a utilitarian approach that uses income and wealth to assess the standard of living in one country, it proposes the definition of development as an expansion of 'capabilities' that lead people to flourish. The Capability Approach differentiates capabilities from functioning. The latter refers to the 'being' and 'doing' of a person, while the former refers to the 'substantive freedom' that a person has to achieve their desired functioning. Functioning reflects a person's actual achievements, while the capability set 'represents the freedom to achieve: the alternative functioning combinations from which this person can choose' (Sen, 1999: 75).

From this viewpoint mental health can be understood as a state of flourishing, a state of well-being one would want to achieve. It is also a capability as it facilitates achievement of functioning in other aspects of life and the deprivation of this capability will lead to other capability deprivations. An example could be dropping out of school as a result of a mental health crisis and persistent symptoms that make concentration to read difficult. As Ariana and Naveed put it, because of the 'intrinsic and instrumental role' of health in achieving well-being, 'lack of health can therefore be the heart of inter-locking deprivations', resulting in multiple deprivation (2009: 239).

I identified five reasons for using the Capabilities Approach as a theoretical framework, which provide an evaluative element into a structural approach to recovery. First, capabilities as substantive freedom is based on the values of the Capabilities Approach seeing agency as the basis for achieving flourishing or well-being (Hopper, 2007; Davidson *et al.*, 2009). Substantive freedom consists of two dimensions: process and opportunities. As Sen states, 'processes that allow freedom of actions and decision, and the actual opportunities that people have, given their personal and social circumstance' (1999: 17). The 'process' dimension resonates with the rights-based recovery that asserts service users' rights to choose, or self-determination. As Davidson *et al.*, put it,

> it is crucially important within this framework to understand that freedom is not a 'thing' (i.e. a resource) that one person can give *to* or establish *for* another. Rather, it becomes incumbent on the first party, morally and practically, to afford the second party opportunities to make his or her own choices (of what to do and be) and to determine his or her own fate.
>
> (2009: 40)

It does not only call for positive risk-taking, but also a scrutiny of the possible mistreatment and intervention that strips service users of self-determination.

Thus the Capabilities Approach can provide the principle of a policy framework and because of its emphasis on human rights it can be potentially used with existing human rights legislative frameworks at national and international levels (Carpenter, 2009b; Wallcraft and Hopper, 2015). This 'process' aspect of capabilities also suggests a collective level of participation. As discussed in Chapter 1, recovery is perceived by service user advocates as no longer a service user led agenda in the UK. Supporting people to recovery should not be about pre-setting their path as implied in the government's 'welfare to work' programmes. The outcome of recovery is evaluated not by what the people actually choose to do, but by what capabilities (exercisable freedom to choose one's valued life) are expanded. Therefore, in this book, instead of using the term 'successful recovery', I use 'meaningful recovery', i.e. recovery with goals that are meaningful to service users themselves.

The Capabilities Approach takes account of social influences and scope for exercising agency in a number of ways. Self-determination is meaningless if there is no alternative that one can choose from. The Capabilities Approach is not concerned with what a person's actual choices are. This is where the opportunities dimension of capabilities fits in. According to Hopper (2007: 874), 'what one chooses is less important than the range of valued options actually entertained, developmentally available and socially sanctioned'. The emphasis on a range of valued options directly critiques the 'pseudo-choice', which is involved when a service user is only allowed to 'voluntarily' or 'involuntary' admit themselves to hospital, because there are no service alternatives such as home treatment crisis teams. It also challenges the neo-liberal consumerist discourse of users' choice that ignores the contraction of the available treatment and service options that can be chosen because of financial cuts to health and welfare under 'austerity', as is happening in the UK. Recovery progress can be understood as an opportunities gradient (Hopper, 2007). Opportunities here do not just refer to the range of service options. They include at a macro level life chances in the hierarchical social structure.

Second, the Capabilities Approach provides a basis for developing a social model of mental health with political leverage, like the social model of disability for disability rights. The applicability of the social model of disability to mental health has been debated at length in the literature (Spandler *et al.*, 2015). The social model of disability draws a distinction between individual impairment and disability, arguing that impairment leads to a disabling experience because of the social barriers, discrimination and oppression, not as a direct result of the impairment itself (Beresford, 2002). For example, The notion of 'recovery in' proposed by Davidson and his colleagues is to call for a social model of disability that moves attention away from treatment to ensuring that service users have a quality of life. Living with persistent symptoms that may or may not result in a poor quality of life and compromised community living depends on the environment lived in (Davidson *et al.*, 2005; Davidson and Roe, 2007).

In the UK, the mental health service user movement is aware of the importance of alliances with the disabled people's movement, because psychiatric illness is positioned under the same 'pathologising administrative category' that move people into a 'sick role' to access entitlements for support and welfare. So both groups experience the impact of labelling and stigma. However, many mental health service users do not feel comfortable being identified as disabled and do not feel impaired (Beresford, 2000, 2002, Beresford *et al.*, 2012). Such reactions are not simply a subjective rejection of stigma, but relate to the drawbacks of the social model of disability, which may not be able to capture the subtleties and complexities of the relationship between the actual impairment and the wider social environment (Shakespeare, 2007; Thomas, 2008; cited in Wallcraft and Hopper, 2015). Mitra (2006) argues that the focus of exercisable opportunities in the Capabilities Approach allows for an analysis of the interaction among individual characteristics, resources available and the environment.

This is particularly relevant to the controversy in mental health about whether psychiatric diagnoses, such as 'personality disorder', are a pathology or a difference. This connects to the point Fernando (2009) raised about recovery. In response to the question 'what does one recover from if not illness?' (Fernando, 2009: 23) he argues that an emphasis on 'recovery' from 'care' reinforces Western ways of thinking. He proposes to balance the concepts of 'liberation' and 'therapy', in which the former implies liberation from 'problems or suffering'. The Capabilities Approach can help evaluate how a deprivation in mental well-being leads to multiple deprivations in different aspects of life, resulting in a downward movement along the opportunity gradient, without a need to pathologies suffering. It can also help evaluate the usefulness of certain interventions, adjustments to the immediate environment, and policies if they can redevelop enhance or extend the capabilities deprivation linked to 'impairment', 'suffering' or 'difference' (whatever service users understand their conditions to be).

Third, the Capabilities Approach is sensitive to diversity and multiculturalism, because of its concern with whether one has economic and political opportunities in place to choose one's valued way of life, instead of what one choses eventually (Nussbaum, 2000). This view rejects the notion of 'assimilation' for ethnic minorities or 'going back to work' for mental health service users as the only socially accepted goal of recovery. A structural approach to recovery in relation to members of ethnic minorities, would view social inclusion as ensuring that ethnic minorities have the capabilities to live in the ways they want to live, be it the same or different from the mainstream.

Carpenter (2009b) proposes combining the Capabilities Approach and the discussion of extensive economic and social rights (ESC) to provide a single frame of holistic analysis focused on people's needs and entitlements. Using the Capabilities Approach and the Equality Review, Carpenter argues, can potentially combine what Fraser (1995) has termed the 'politics of redistribution' and 'politics of recognition' (see also Robeyns, 2003), as well as avoiding an exclusionary version of citizenship based on national identity (hence resulting in capabilities deprivation). For example, 'justice', 'equality' and 'fairness' can be judged by comparing the opportunity gradient of different disadvantaged and privileged groups.

Taking this approach, the Chinese in the UK as well as mental health service users face double disadvantages. In fact, it can be multi-dimensional inequality that a Chinese mental health service user experiences if they face class inequality, gender oppression and ageism at the same time. At a policy level, this prompts the question of whether subsuming different equalities into a single policy and institutional framework can deal with the intersecting characteristics of inequalities or risk diluting the strength of existing mechanisms such as gender mainstreaming (Kantola and Squires, 2010).

Applying this, in this study, involves finding out how service users' capabilities have changed throughout their recovery journeys, and then analysing the types of inequalities, if any, that have resulted in capabilities deprivation. In addition a Capabilities Approach that pays attention to diversity enables a discussion of what capabilities are considered important for a particular group, as well as addressing diversity inside the group. It is helpful in attending to the heterogeneity within Chinese communities.

Fourth, the discussion so far about the use of the Capabilities Approach in mental health resonates with Strength Models (Rapp, 1998) and social capital theory (McKenzie *et al.*, 2002). They share commonalities in terms of their emphasis on the material, social and cultural resources one owns and advocates for the development of these resources. Yet, Prilleltensky (2005) shows that a singular focus on strengths and empowerment is not enough for achieving well-being. For interventions in promoting well-being, fostering individual skills need to go hand in hand with tackling damaging community conditions. The Capabilities Approach argues that one's resources do not necessarily convert into capabilities. For example, a desired 'doing' such as a competent applicant applying for a job, may encounter discrimination because of their past psychiatric history.

Therefore, the development of the applicant's capabilities is dependent on 'conversion factors', e.g. the existence of anti-discrimination legislation. 'Conversion factors' can be personal, social and environmental (Robeyns, 2005). As for mental well-being as a desired state of 'being', health inequalities are closely related to educational level, social status, occupational hierarchy and family dynamics (Ariana and Naveed, 2009). Conversion factors determine how steep an individual's opportunities gradient is i.e. the relative difficulties individuals experience in capabilities development. Thus, the notion of conversion factors show that the outcomes of education, retraining, or rehabilitation programmes that are designed to develop capabilities result in different outcomes because the input of resources is the same for a heterogeneous group of people. Therefore, in linking with discussions of diversity and evaluating what hinders or facilitates capabilities development, it is important to analyse the role of different conversion factors. For example, the role of cultural difference needs to be examined when considering the benefits of home treatment for Chinese mental health service users.

Finally, the Capabilities Approach can provide a critique of the consumerist view of choice with its notion of adaptive preference. A utilitarian view of choice or satisfaction does not take into account how an individual's preference is adaptive to the social structure. The Capabilities Approach puts preference under scrutiny to reveal 'the many ways in which habit, fear, low expectations, and unjust background conditions deform people's choices and even their wishes for their own lives' (Nussbaum, 2000: 114). Wallcraft found that adaptive preferences are often revealed in the quality of life studies that compare the reduced quality of life using 'objective' measures with the responses given by service users, the latter tend to 'minimise their losses' (Wallcraft, 2010; 2011).

This has resonance with the discussion of 'false consciousness', which some may consider patronising. However, as Deneulin, puts it, to understand adaptive preference is 'not a question of identifying those whose capabilities have been deformed as against "free" individuals, but of accepting that all are subject to restraints and conditioning which affect how they exercise their choices'

(2008: 118). Adaptive preference can be distinguished from 'revealed preference' because the former comprises capability development (Nussbaum, 2000; Unterhalter, 2009). This has a number of implications for researching recovery. Questions need to be asked about the self-reporting of satisfaction in understanding service users' needs and aspiration. When hope is explored it should be remembered that asking service users about their goals of recovery may generate a response that reflects a lowered aspiration due to the avoidance of disappointment and frustration because of repeated experiences of invalidation in the past (Hopper, 2007).

Questions need to be asked about worldview and life aspiration in order to understand revealed preference. It is also important to reveal the conversion factors that result in lowered aspiration through scrutinising how adaptive preference is formed along the recovery journey. In the case of ethnic minorities, direct experience of discrimination and perceived discrimination can be a barrier to social inclusion, limiting the range of opportunities that a service user gauges they should 'sensibly' expect.

Finally, the lowered aspiration may actually reveal social inequalities and hardships. The popularisation of encouraging 'positive thinking' without tackling the real problems of the social environment service users live in, risk rendering 'hope' and 'positive thinking' as an ideology that displaces the necessity of collective structural changes to individual adjustment problems that reinforce self-blame (Ehrenreich, 2010).

In sum, while the Capabilities Approach builds upon the premise of the importance of agency in enabling an individual's capability development, an explicit assessment about the 'structure of living together' is important (Deneulin, 2008). As discussed above, the opportunities dimension of capabilities one has is dependent on what is sanctioned by the opportunities structure of society. Sayer (2012) argues for an examination of social structure to account for what enables or restricts capabilities, using job shortage and the unequal division of labour as examples of external determinants that restrict capabilities. For example, in relation to understanding the social inclusion of Chinese mental health service users, it is important to analyse the social mobility structure and the segmented labour market experienced by the Chinese in the UK.

'Agency is not a tabula rasa, but is itself the produce of certain structures of living together' (Deneulin, 2008: 120). The subjective meaning one has is foregrounded by these structures. In fact, Deneulin proposes to understand agency as 'socio-historical', i.e. choices an individual makes are crucially dependent on the socio-historical structures they are positioned in. An examination of the socio-historical structure of living together, the external conditions of capabilities, is thus vital to examining the preconditions for individuals to exercise choice. Intersectionality Analysis is employed for this investigation.

Intersectionality Analysis and social location

While the Capabilities Approach provides a heuristic tool to track capabilities development along the recovery journey, Intersectionality Analysis can be used to delineate what enables or hinders capabilities development and analyses the role of conversion factors in terms of generative mechanisms and power relations. Intersectionality Analysis allows for enquiry into the interplay of structure and agency and how it plays out in relation to the complexity of inequality and diversity and their variability in people's lives.

Intersectionality studies emerged from feminist studies, arising from criticisms against the failure of second wave feminism to recognise diversity in women's experiences when advancing solidarity claims for women's rights (e.g. Crenshaw, 1991; Collins, 1998; McCall, 2005). The concern of intersectionality studies to avoid a simplistic additive way of understanding the effect of different dimensions of social inequalities such as class, gender, race, by exploring the social and historical processes of how they intersect and mutually shape each other, resulting in particular experiences of oppression. It has been mainly used in research with an explicit feminist perspective but is a transferable method of analysis that has the potential to deepen understandings of how different forms of oppression are experienced in relation to a range of social inequalities (e.g. Choo and Ferree, 2010).

This study on Chinese communities in the UK is akin to what Choo and Ferree (2010) classified as 'inclusion-centered interpretations' that give voices to the marginalised and show the effects of multiple inequalities. However, Choo and Ferree (2010) warn about the danger of 'fetish-ing' the 'differences', going against the original intention to avoid essentialising cultural differences, which may result from lack of 'structural analysis of how distinctive ways of life are created in, and for, a wider system of class, race and gender privilege' (Choo and Ferree, 2010: 138). To avoid this they suggest problematising the mainstream explicitly in the analysis, e.g. by examining 'how the more powerful are defined as normative standards' (Choo and Ferree, 2010: 133).

The danger of 'fetish-ing' 'differences' can also be a result of foregrounding one or two dimensions of inequalities in the analysis while treating others such as class, gender and age as demographic background factors (van Mens-Verhulst and Radtke, 2008). While 'ethnic inequalities' is one dimension to explore in this study of members of an ethnic minority group, I would not assume a priori that other power or inequality dimensions are less important in contributing to mental health capabilities deprivation or hindering the (re)development of capabilities along the recovery journey. Because of the heterogeneity within Chinese communities, it is anticipated that a variety of recovery journeys will be found among Chinese service users as they are subject to a variety of ways that structural forces impact on them. For this reason, from the interview with service users I aimed to find out the 'social location' of each service user and then explore the systems of inequality at play in shaping that social location.

A critical realist conceptualisation of 'intersectionality' and 'social location' is used in this study. Walby *et al.* (2012) propose using unequal social relations as the focus of analysis without losing sight of the actions of the powerful and the structures and understandings that different social relations play in 'mutually shaping' each other. Anthias' argument (2006) about conceptualising social location as 'translocational positionality' is particularly relevant to this study. In relation to the 'translocational', she claims that global and transnational context is significant in understanding how ethnic inequality is manifested at the local level. Survival strategies can be dependent on the globalised network. This is not just relevant for sojourners, but also those locally born and long settled migrants. If sense of belonging is a quality of life, or in the terms used in the Capabilities Approach's a valued 'functioning', Anthias argues that this is not just about geographical boundaries but also 'hierarchies that exist both within and cut across boundaries' (2006: 22), for the differential inclusions and exclusions based on gender, ethnicity, class, age, and for this study, psychiatric power, sanism and ableism. Understanding 'social location' as 'positionality' thus combines 'a reference to social position (as a set of effectiveness, or as outcome) and social positioning (as a set of practices, actions and meanings, as process)' (Anthias 2001: 634, quoted in Anthias 2006: 27). Positionality denotes the social hierarchy (opportunities structure, local as well as transnational) and agency (meaning and practice) and connects with the Capabilities Approach in using capabilities as the evaluative space.

Investigating the positionality of the individuals or groups can thus help us explore how misery, madness and incorrigibility *as well as* the subsequent deviance are produced. The exclusionary force service users experience started before social reactions to their display of distress or incorrigible practices such as public prejudice or medical labelling. The cumulative effect of the oppression or exclusionary forces from various inequalities makes one vulnerable to distress and mental ill health. Thus, situating the practice of misery and 'madness' with one's positionality can help us trace and explore the generative mechanisms that produce them in the first place. For example, research on the traumagenic neurodevelopmental model offers one set of generative mechanisms to explain psychotic symptoms with adverse life events such as childhood trauma and poverty (Read, 2010; Read and Bentall, 2012). Humiliation and a sense of entrapment, which are markers of unequal social relations, were linked to risk of depression in women (Brown *et al.*, 1995). To understand this with 'labelling' theory (Scheff, 1966), primary deviance is the practices that arise from psychological "disturbance' or 'impairment' that might result from difficult circumstances and the actions of others (e.g. poor parenting, prolonged exploitation or entrapment). Secondary deviance thus occurred when these practices of misery and 'madness' were labelled by public and medical professionals as problematic or intelligible due to 'rule transgression' or 'infraction' that has normative implications (Pilgrim and Tomasini, 2012). Here, positionality reflects what set of classed, gendered or ethnicised ideologies were deemed to be violated, resulting in labelling and exclusion to 'contain' these perceived 'deviant' behaviours or practices. This is where ableism and sanism intersects with other inequalities to emerge as another set of generative mechanisms that can impede (re)development of capabilities, restrict one's life chances and subsequently position one even further down the social hierarchy.

Towards a synthesis of the Capabilities Approach and Intersectionality Analysis

How are the Capabilities Approach and Intersectionality Analysis used in guiding the empirical exploration of the interplay of agency and structure in this study? To research what Chinese people with received diagnoses recover from and into becomes an exploration of the way their capabilities set change over the recovery journey. As we shall see in the following chapters, the ebb and flow of their recovery journeys can be reflected in terms of capability changes. Capabilities loss and deprivation is what limits an individual's coping resources and contributes to mental ill health and distress. Using the metaphor from the Tidal model, the interplay of the structural forces of class, gender, ethnicity contribute to people 'drowning' because of their mental distress and capabilities loss (Barker and Bachunan-Barker, 2005).

These structural forces intersect with psychiatric power, sanism and abelism in changing the life chances the service users have along their recovery journeys. What they recover from, which this study asks, is thus what capabilities are lost or deprived to achieve individuals' valued 'doings' and beings'. Meaningful recovery is then a (re)development of capabilities to live a desired life. While one's capability is (re)developed along the recovery journey, it is possible that another capability can be lost at different phases of the journey. A move from patienthood to personhood would entail an expansion of multidimensional capabilities.

In relation to agency, the extent that individuals have the capabilities, or 'substantial freedom' to engage in actions and choices to realise their valued 'beings' and 'doings' will be explored in this book. Capabilities or substantial freedom have two dimensions, process and opportunities. In this study, as will be shown in the subsequent chapters, the process dimension involves researching decision-making processes in making life choices as well as during changes in the recovery journey. It explores whether these act as restrictions to exercising agency, for example, violations of human rights and their contribution to mental distress and ill health. Whether an individual's life decisions or choices relating to seeking help from health and social services are self-determining, or are adaptive preferences due to lack of viable options or alternatives. The way Chinese service users make sense and reflect on their recovery journeys, the life strategies they employ to achieve desired 'doings' and 'beings, the way their hope and life goals change over the recovery journey are explored in relation to their past experiences, current capabilities set and perceived social opportunities in the future.

Regarding the opportunities side of capability, the variations of social locations of Chinese service users in the UK provide entry points to understanding the different exercisable opportunities they have to achieve their valued 'beings' and 'doings'. Understanding social location in terms of translocational positionality, these exercisable opportunities, or life chances, are a result of the intersection of different structural forces that constitute the intra- and trans-national social hierarchies the service user is positioned in. Their biographies could be understood as 'translocational life histories'.

How different structural forces constitute barriers or provide opportunities for capability development can be mutually reinforcing or contradictory (Anthias, 2006). This can result in a smaller capabilities set and steeper opportunities gradient. The effect of diminished capability in one area of life may be softened by capability in another area. In turn, identities in relation to structural forces such as class, gender, ethnicity, sanism and ableism may inform the strategies Chinese service users employ to make sense of and strive to work towards a meaningful recovery. This interplay of structure and agency is captured in the following chapters through their journeys of recovery.

3 When things start to fall apart

Social conditions and the loss of capabilities

Introduction

This chapter introduces the participants and presents data from their narratives about what they considered they were recovering from. The aim of this chapter is to expand understandings of what recovery from 'symptoms' (in the clinical model) and 'social skills' (in the rehabilitative model) means. It explores the capabilities that were important to the mental well-being of the participant's prior to their mental health deterioration. It also provides a critical analysis of the socio-structural conditions that contributed to their distress and ill health in the first place.

In the next section of this chapter, the participants are positioned in relation to the social history of Chinese communities in the UK. An assessment of their capabilities sets, in particular the life chances they had at different points in their life histories, is made. A background is given, so that their biographies and predicaments are given a context.

Then I will discuss what led to the participants reaching crisis point because of a deterioration in their mental health. The social conditions in which deterioration occurred and the role played by structural inequalities is considered. The relationship between the positioning of participants and the processes leading to the diminishing of their mental health capabilities is organised around seven key themes that emerged from their narratives. These were:

- citizenship and the position of undocumented migrants;
- developing capabilities in education;
- Chinese in the UK labour market and the working conditions in the Chinese catering business;
- overseas brides;
- informal caring work;
- childbirth;
- aging and isolation.

The social conditions that the participants needed to recover from and how the intersectionality of class, gender and ethnicity played out in shaping these social conditions is also analysed.

The names of the participants here are pseudonyms, apart from Raymond who wanted to keep his real name as, he said, there was nothing to be ashamed of in disclosing his recovery story.

Positioning the service users

The 13 female and 9 male service users who participated in this research were spread across age groups (Table 3.1) and places of birth (Table 3.2). Two service users had been born in the UK, the other 20 were born in mainland China, Hong Kong or Vietnam.

The commonalities and differences among the male and female participants were characterised by their different life stages as well as their geographical locales prior to coming to the UK. Their narratives revealed their gendered life courses in terms of gendered patterns of work and family and the influence of gender ideologies in the formation of adaptive and revealed preferences in their life goals and plans. The articulation of the gendered ideologies about normative life course that are loaded into 'Chinese' cultures varies according to the societies they had lived in. For example, the so-called 'prime time' for woman to get married in mainland China was younger than that for women in Hong Kong. Subsequent chapters trace the effects of gender ideology and structure on the participants. However, it cannot be assumed that normative gender ideologies are followed by default. Moving to the UK, for some, deliberately or not, was a way to distance themselves from social norms that were experienced as sources of pressure.

An overarching theme that emerged from the participants' narratives was the significance of transnational context in understanding the social conditions that foster or hinder the development of capabilities contributive to mental well-being. This applies to both the migrants in this study and the second generation Chinese who were born in the UK. The transmission of cultural values by first-generation parents and the common practice for second-generation members to be sent to Chinese school to learn Chinese language skills were important. The family network of their parents in their place of origin, temporary reserve

Table 3.1 Age and gender of the participants at the time of interview

	<30	31–40	41–50	51–60	60+
Female	0	6	1	4	3
Male	3	0	3	0	2

Table 3.2 Birthplace of participants

	UK	Mainland China	Hong Kong	Vietnam
Female	0	6	6	1
Male	2	1	6	0

migration, the circulation of values and beliefs in popular culture via information technology were all ways that the second generation maintained a foot in the 'Chinese world' outside the UK.

Becoming an ethnic minority: Chinese communities in the UK and the biographies of participants

The ways ethnicity shaped social locations were marked by the different ways participants 'became' ethnic minorities in the UK. The year the participants migrated into the UK ranged from 1966 to 2010, reflecting the population movement of Chinese people into the UK over different periods of time. Chinese settlement in the UK started as early as the nineteenth century when Chinese men were employed as seamen. Between World War II and the 1950s Chinese immigrants were mostly from South East Asia. Hong Kong was a colony of UK from 1841 to 1997. The late 1950s saw a wave of Chinese immigration to the UK from Hong Kong. This was mostly of young males from rural areas in Hong Kong. The worsening economic conditions they faced in Hong Kong at that time was partly a result of the political interest of the UK colonial government in developing Hong Kong as a trading port for English firms rather than a sustainable economy for the needs of rural residents (Yu, 2000). Several male participants came to the UK from this background.

Other political reasons for immigration included the hand over of Hong Kong from UK to China in 1997. Worry about the unclear future under the rule of the Communist Party, led many people to migrate to other countries, including the UK. Carol's husband migrated to the UK for this reason. During the colonial era, Hong Kong was the port of 'first asylum' for refugees fleeing the Vietnam War. Refugees would then seek asylum to European countries. Rachel came from Vietnam via Hong Kong when she was a baby. Migration from mainland China has risen in recent years because of relaxations in emigration controls since 1985 (Kagan *et al.*, 2011). China's economic growth has meant that a fast growing number of people who can afford to travel, study abroad and have migrated to other countries.

Migration could be framed or defined as an anticipated capabilities development process for migrants in this study. The reasons they migrated, the experience of the migration process and settling in the UK reflected their life chances in their homeland as well as the opportunities they had expected in the UK. Immigration policies as well as experienced and anticipated racial discrimination in the UK at different periods of time facilitated and constrained migration as a capabilities development process.

From the 1960s to the 1970s, the decline of agricultural industry in Hong Kong as well as the right granted to live and work in the UK coincided with a rise in the demand for Chinese catering in the UK. This resulted in the establishment of Chinese catering businesses as a familial strategy for migration and capability development. These catering businesses were usually family run with family members providing cheap labour in order to increase the competitiveness of the business (Baxter, 1988).

Lai-Ming migrated to the UK from Hong Kong in the 1960s with his family hoping to improve the family's economic condition. As a young man he was offered a place at university. At that time, Hong Kong's higher education participation rate was less than 10 per cent (Wu, 2008). Going to university was restricted to the privileged because of the high tuition fees. Although Lai-Ming had academic ability, his working-class family could not afford the fees. Instead of going to university, he passed the examination to become a civil servant. Working as a civil servant during this time was considered to be an 'iron rice bowl' because of its job security and pension (Hong Kong does not have a universal pension scheme). Lai-Ming's parental family decided to come to the UK to run a restaurant business. The business was not successful and Lai-Ming had to then find work in other Chinese restaurants.

For many of the female migrant participants, marriage was the reason to come to the UK. They were usually from lower-class backgrounds. Eight female participants migrated to the UK to marry settled Chinese migrants. However, not all female migrants migrated to the UK because of marriage. Lee *et al.* (2002) investigated the migration strategies of Chinese women. They found that apart from marrying Chinese migrants or White British men, women were also independent migrants who came to the UK for individual advancement such as education or training.

Coming to the UK for individual advancement as independent migrants has become increasingly popular in recent years. The expansion of the UK higher education market's recruitment of overseas students has come together with the rapidly growing economy of mainland China. This has meant that the super rich as well as the growing middle classes have the economic power to seek education and training overseas. Many of them are also interested in seeking opportunities to stay in the UK to work. Hins, who came to the UK in 2010, was a participant who reflected this trajectory.

Marriage as an institution is worth further exploration for the way it intersects with the social hierarchy of Chinese lower-class families in the UK as well as that of lower-class families in Chinese societies. Chinese families in the UK might go to their hometown in mainland China to find suitable brides for their sons. Men who had spent most of their time in family catering businesses, can find it difficult to socialise and find potential marriage partners themselves. The prejudice and discrimination found in Chinese communities against other ethnic minorities means that the incidence of intercultural marriage with other ethnicities is low. The disadvantage faced by Chinese men in the UK marriage market was compensated for in extending the search for brides to their Chinese hometowns. It was a common anticipation among migrants, that life in an advanced industrial country like the UK would be better than life in a small rural town in mainland China. For the family of the bride, as the narratives of participants showed, arranging for a daughter to marry overseas was considered to be a way for her to move up the social ladder and secure a better livelihood. However, as subsequent chapters show, this path for capabilities development in which the bride depended on the groom's family could result in capability deprivation.

This does not mean that all overseas brides were held captive by their in-laws. However, the opportunities and agency of overseas brides could be compromised through this form of marriage.

Participants who had been born or raised in the UK from their earliest years were members of an ethnic minority whose life chances were heavily influenced by the migration history of their parents. Their parents' economic and social capital as well as their aspirations could have an impact on the capabilities development of participants growing up in the UK. The deprivation of capabilities set, in terms of economic support and social networks, could have an adverse impact on mental health as Rachel and Jerry's narratives illustrated.

Socio-economic status and language skills as part of capabilities sets

The socio-economic position and the language skills of the participants reflected the capabilities sets they had in living a life they wanted, working in a satisfying job with decent pay, living in locations they liked and accessing the health and social care services they needed. However these resources and abilities constitute only part of capabilities sets for two reasons. First, whether they could be converted into exercisable opportunities depend on the structural and institutional arrangement of a society. Second, whether a low ability or low income is a capability deprivation is dependent on the context. For example, low English language skills can be a capability deprivation in terms of accessing public services only when there is no interpretation service provided to ensure equality of access.

The aim of reflecting on the partial capabilities set here is to help understand the opportunities gradients the participants were positioned on. This therefore enables us to evaluate the social conditions that one recovered from, i.e. what helps or hinders the (re)development of the participants' mental health and other related capabilities along their recovery journeys. Occupation is a key indicator of one's socio-economic position. The work histories of participants in the UK were gendered (Table 3.3).

Table 3.3 Occupations of participants in the UK

'Helping out' in family-run takeaways	2 (women)
University teaching	1 (woman)
Personal assistant in an elderly care home	1 (woman)
Waiting staff at Chinese restaurants	4 (men)
Part-time cleaner	1 (man)
Printing factory	1 (man)
Bank	1 (man)
IT-related management	1 (man)
Design	1 (man)
Laboratory	1 (man)
Waiting staff at a hotel	1 (man)

At the time of interview, none of the participants were holding a full-time job. Two were full-time students. One woman had a contractual part-time job as personal assistant in an elderly care home and one man was working part-time in a Chinese restaurant.

Chapter 5 explores how many participants experienced downward occupational mobility along the recovery process, with an accompanying diminishment of work capability. Occupational mobility is strongly related to an individual's educational level. Table 3.4 shows participants' educational levels. Several participants had to drop out of university because of a mental health breakdown and were unable to go back to their studies. The role of educational institutions in capability development and the environment that is counter-contributive to mental well-being will be discussed further in the next section of this chapter.

As shown in Table 3.5, more than half of the participants lived in public housing and two participants lived in supported housing. Housing type reflects an individual's socioeconomic status, as well as the type of neighbourhood lived in.

One indicator of ethnic difference and inequalities is language ability. Not being able to speak English fluently is one major reason for not being able to participate extensively in UK life or make friends outside the Chinese community. Table 3.6 shows the participants' language skills.

All the participants who were only fluent in Chinese languages (12 out of 22 participants) said that they would like to improve their English so that they could be independent and not have to rely on other people in order to travel to places and use services. This meant that they found language ability crucial in

Table 3.4 Educational levels of participants

Primary school or below	8
Equivalent to UK Year 9	2
GCSE	2
A-level	5
Further education	2
Higher education	3

Table 3.5 Types of housing of participants at the time of interview

Council housing/housing association	12
Hostel/supported housing	2
Private rental	4
Home ownership by parents or partner	4

Table 3.6 Languages spoken fluently by participants

English only	1
English and Chinese language(s)	9
Chinese language only	12
(e.g. Mandarin and Cantonese)	

exercising their agency. They could converse in day-to-day situations such as shopping with simple English. Sometimes they could manage with their basic vocabularies when seeing a doctor for regular check-ups. They could connect with English-speaking people with simple words, gestures and tones. However, in more complicated situations, for example, a mental health crisis that required articulation of feelings and perhaps the assertion of rights, limitations in English language skills could be experienced as a barrier to empowerment.

All of these participants had attended English courses run by Chinese community centres. However, participants who had heavy caring duties, such as Abao and Bai-Xin, and those who had to be flexible in coping with their persistent symptoms, like Carol, found it difficult to spare time to attend English courses regularly. Even if they did attend courses, they found it difficult to find the time or concentration to revise course material and practice. Many of them had dropped out of English classes as a result.

A glimpse into perceived discrimination

How did the positioning of the participants outlined above, impact on their perceptions of racial discrimination in the UK? Their narratives reflected the variety of ways racial discrimination was perceived and experienced over the years. Individuals did not need to experience a direct racial attack to feel excluded. Ken arrived in the UK in the late 1970s, when he was nearly 20 years old, to pursue a university degree. He said he did not experience direct racist attacks, but he was acutely aware of being 'Other' because of the looks he got from the local people.

> Racial discrimination has always been there. But I have not received much . . . When I lived in Kent many years ago, there were not many Chinese people. I went for a drink in a café, people looked at me like I was a monster. I remember that scenario very well.

This vivid memory reflects Ken's sudden 'realisation' of perceived difference, the attainment of a prescribed 'minority', if not 'alien' status, as a migrant. Around the same time, during the 1980s, Rachel recalled having to move home to avoid racist attacks. She had grown up in the UK, and had been living in London. The neighbourhood she lived in as a child during the 1980s, she recalled as being 'racist'. Overt racist attacks were experienced on the streets. Her parents moved away to protect the family. Rachel was also told by her parents to stop playing outside the family house.

> There used to be a lot of racism where I used to live. A very White area. This area I am living now is very White too, but it's not racist here. In the old area, we were told to stay inside. We ignored those people.

Like Rachel's family, Ken felt he 'blended' in after relocation. He moved to North London and felt at ease there.

I felt that I was not living in Britain, because it's not easy to find a White British there. Not on the bus or on the street. Especially in the fitness club. I can hardly find a White British. Mostly Polish and others. So I felt that I was not living in Britain! . . . It was very multicultural. Very metropolitan. This is one of the reasons I like London. There isn't much overt discrimination.

While at school, Rachel could feel subtle undercurrents. 'I won't say there is no racism. But I think it's out of school there is a lot. I think in school the teachers are there, so it's ok.'

Rachel pointed out the important role of teachers in tackling bullying and racism. Being able to trust teacher's readiness to tackle racist bullying seemed to be key for participants to feel protected from racism in school and hence not to be compromised in pursuing educational opportunities in a safe environment.

Ken liked the multicultural environment in the capital city. However, he seemed to think that racial discrimination in the workplace was unavoidable. His view that racial discrimination is a given fact no matter which ethnic group one belongs to is quite common among members of Chinese communities. 'Like working . . . of course you don't want to be discriminated at work. But I won't be surprised to find a certain dosage of racial discrimination. Like Chinese people also discriminate against others.'

Ken's views were expressed in others participants' narratives. Alongside direct racial attacks on a day-to-day basis, the participants experienced disadvantages, as the result of racism, at a structural level as subsequent chapters will show.

Capabilities loss: social conditions and the deterioration of mental well-being

The last section provided a background of the migration trajectories of the service users or that of their parents, and the positioning of the service users in the social hierarchy in terms of social class, ethnicity and gender. This section focuses on the social conditions that contributed to the deterioration of participants' mental health, leading to crisis point. How class, ethnicity and gender intersected and the ways they expanded or contracted the participants' capabilities will be analysed.

The seven themes that emerged from the analysis of the narratives related to common social conditions shared by some of the participants. They also highlighted how a set of social conditions could limit an individual's capability.

Citizenship: undocumented migrants

Citizenship status is a crucial determinant of an individual's capability set to access the labour market as well as health and social care entitlements. At the time of the interviews, 20 of the participants had UK permanent residency and 2 had student visas. Feng entered the UK illegally, sought asylum and was granted permanent residency later. The changes in immigration policies in the UK reflect international relations, the domestic economy and the anti-immigration climate within the country.

As the UK allows citizens to hold dual citizenship, migrants who came from a country that also permits citizens to hold dual citizenship would have more choice, hence more capabilities, than others if they wanted to go back to their homeland. They would also be able to access public services and welfare exclusive to citizens in their home country. Since mainland China does not allow dual citizenship, migrants from mainland China could not easily return to China if their lives do not work out for them in the UK. Hong Kong permits emigrants to keep their Hong Kong citizenship. Participants who came from Hong Kong and had obtained British citizenship therefore enjoyed dual citizenship.

Raymond was born in the UK but had moved with his family and lived in Hong Kong for a few years. Ken had then migrated to the UK and obtained UK citizenship long before his first breakdown. Following his family's migration to the UK, he had been thinking of going back to Hong Kong for work as he thought that Hong Kong would be more 'exciting'. With dual citizenship he was able to reside in both Hong Kong and the UK. Going between UK and Hong Kong was an integral component of his recovery journey after his breakdown. Carol said she too had considered moving back to Hong Kong after her mental health crisis.

The capability set of an asylum seeker, like Feng, is low compared with the various kinds of residency status held by the other participants. Before applying for asylum status, Feng could only work illegally and could not access statutory health and welfare services. Feng came to the UK from a fishing village in mainland China in 2000 when he was 20. With only a primary school education, Feng's chances of making a good living in his home village was small. As a result of the unequal development between rural and urban areas in mainland China since its Open Door policy was introduced in 1978, many young adults migrated to cities to look for work opportunities. Undocumented migration to the UK was a way for Feng to, in his words, 'explore the world'. His girlfriend, who later became his wife, had gone to the UK before him. He did not plan to stay for good nor did he anticipate applying for asylum. He just wanted to work and bring money home. He was mindful of keeping a low profile in case he was caught by the immigration services. But he expressed indifference about the possibility of getting arrested. He found the harsh working conditions in Chinese restaurants and the pressure of starting a family when his girlfriend became pregnant more distressing and pressing than his worries about being repatriated.

Having helped his fisherman father in China until he was 20, moving to a big UK city to work in Chinese restaurants was a huge change for Feng. The burden of supporting a family was a pressure for him. Living as an undocumented immigrant, hidden and feeling as if he were at the bottom of a foreign society, he had very limited capability in making provision for his family. It was manageable when he lived alone. However, with a child coming soon, the limited capability set he and his wife had meant that life for their household was very difficult.

The below minimum wages he and his wife earned meant it was difficult to provide for their child. His lack of legal citizenship meant that public services were inaccessible. Feng started not being able to, in his words, 'think normally'. His acquaintances were mostly people from his hometown. However, he did not think of asking them for help, as he thought people who went overseas to work were 'self-centred'. He quit his job when his boss started to complain about him becoming introverted.

> My boss got a feeling that . . . he asked my uncle about me. My uncle did not know things about mental health. He asked, 'Why do you look blank all day? Why did you respond so slowly when your boss told you to do things? If you carry on like this, I am sure you can't carry on with the job'. He meant I'd better stop working in this job. Then the boss said things about me and I started having chaotic thoughts.

Feng said he heard voices, got lost on the streets and attempted suicide. Eventually he was sectioned under the Mental Health Act and detained in hospital. He knew some other undocumented migrants whose mental ill health made them decide to go back to China. However, this was not the decision he made. He and his wife had to pay their debt to those who had arranged their passage to the UK. Because his wife thought they needed to earn enough money to do this, she decided to apply for asylum for them to stay in the UK.

Developing capabilities in education

Compared to asylum seekers, participants born in the UK with full citizen rights had a greater opportunity to develop capabilities to work and have social lives because they had been educated in the UK. Participants born in the UK, i.e. second-generation migrants, or those that migrated to the UK with their family at a very young age, had spent their formative years in the UK. One commonality they had was that they experienced a mental health crisis during their higher education studies. They dropped out of study because of this and were unable to return. As Chapter 5 indicates, being unable to obtain educational qualifications because of mental ill health meant that these participants were unable to put their talents to good use in employment.

Rachel attributed her breakdown to the financial stress of doing part-time work while studying at university. Rachel's father passed away when she was a child. Her mother raised six children by working in low-paid jobs with her limited English skills. The lack of financial resources in the family had an adverse impact on Rachel's capability development. Given the financial situation of the family, Rachel worked part-time when studying arts at university. She got a loan for the tuition fees, but she had to earn money to live. Not only did this divert her attention from participating in university life fully, the financial stress took a toll on her mental health. Rachel started to have headaches, she forgot things and places and was not able to recognise her family's faces. At first she thought she was just being 'forgetful'. Later on she started 'seeing relatives' who were dead and found that she could not travel from her home to her university, which was in another city, because she could not remember the route back.

Jerry's narrative reflected the impact of the aspirations of first-generation migrants to see their children being upwardly mobile. This resulted in a struggle for him as a young adult to gain autonomy from parents and the restrictions of the social network of his family. His parents came to the UK in the 1960s, hardly speaking any English. When some missionaries knocked on their door and volunteered to teach them English through the Bible, they welcomed the offer although they had no Christian beliefs. The missionaries became important to Jerry's family as a link to the outside world and provided them with a social network. Jerry's narrative conveyed that the missionaries developed a dominant role in his family. They sowed the seeds of Jerry's deep passion for theology.

Jerry did well in school. He said his parents, who worked as a chef and a bookkeeper, were like other Chinese parents in the UK and wanted him to go to university. They wanted him to graduate and earn good money. However, the leader of the religious group wanted him to become a missionary and did not want him to go to university. Around this time Jerry said he started to suspect that the missionaries were distorting the meaning of the Bible. Jerry said, 'I felt very torn. Very torn'.

He tried to find a middle way between his parents' expectations and the pressure from the missionaries by going to a polytechnic. But he said the missionaries were not pleased with his choice. He suspected that the Christian organisation, which he considered now as a 'sect', was worried that the more education he achieved, the more likely it was that he would challenge their teaching.

It was a difficult situation for Jerry. On the one hand, he felt guilty for upsetting his parents' hopes of him getting a university degree. On the other hand, he wanted to leave the Christian organisation that he realised was a secretive organisation. Although he managed to separate from the missionaries eventually, the feeling of being torn created inner conflicts for him that had a lasting impact. Jerry did not cope well with the first year of independent living at the polytechnic. This was the context in which he had his first psychotic episode.

While the presence of family support meant that Rachel and Jerry were not alone when seeking help from their college medical practice, the help they got was limited as they were not aware of any support, such as counseling, mental health advice or financial assistance that was available to them as students. Rachel was offered a retake of her missed courses. However, she decided to stop her studies because she had become too forgetful and kept getting lost on the journey to university.

These experiences illustrated the importance of universities taking proactive steps to provide flexible support and adjustment for students dealing with mental health problems. Rachel and Jerry studied before the Equality Act (2010) was introduced. This legislation required universities to take up a duty of care for disabled students, including students with mental health problems. In contrast,

Raymond's experience was that support was provided, but its suitability and the way it was offered impacted on his willingness to take it up.

Raymond's narrative was about a series of losses, starting with physical impairment. Having been a promising student, an active athlete and a young man who always rose to challenges and made things happen, the onset of a heart problem changed his life while he was at school. A heart attack resulted in physical impairments that led to speech and memory problems. This all made the organisation of daily life difficult. Raymond moved into supported housing to cope with the aftermath of his heart condition. He was very keen to carry on studying. He went to college but felt that his personal tutor could only help him to a limited extent. When asked if he thought his tutor understood how he could help him he said he didn't think so. He did not make a complaint about his tutor at the time as he thought 'there is only so much the tutor knows and so much he can do'. The college suggested that if he wanted to carry on with his studies he should get a support worker. He rejected this suggestion and had to leave college.

On the surface, it might have been that Raymond was stubborn, which he admitted. However, his narrative reflected the importance of agency. Raymond felt that he was being forced to take up an option. 'I thought it undermined me. If a student wants help he will ask for it. If he wants to go alone and fight every battle with his difficulties he has the right to do that.' He worried that the presence of a support worker would interfere with his socialising,

> Let's change the role. You were me, a shy person, wanting to meet friends but your support is there. Someone comes and talks to your support, and asks him whether they would like to go to a club on Friday night. A person talks to your worker. And you try to join in. The person may think, 'what a rude and unmannered guy'.

Raymond expressed strong feelings about not wanting his agency and dignity compromised. He said his hope to go to university died. He also lost contact with his school friends because he thought they had moved on with their lives. He used to rise to challenges before the heart attack, but now this changed. He could not see possibilities of any improvement and thought of suicide.

Raymond:　I have tried many years, that long now. Just got nothing.
Author:　You feel tired of trying?
Raymond:　I'm not tired. I just think there is no point.

Having to drop out of study shattered the original plans of Jerry, Rachel and Raymond to improve their life chances and realise their aspirations. This not only forced them to review their worldview and life goals but also to reassess what they could do. How their adaptive preferences were developed as a result, i.e. how their outlook and preference in life choice changed in adapting to their predicament, will be discussed further in Chapter 6.

Chinese people in the UK labour market and working conditions in Chinese catering businesses

Employment is an important source of capabilities, but it can also lead to mental ill health that some participants needed to recover from. Many of the participants who had been employed in the UK, had worked in Chinese restaurants. Marcus came to the UK in the 1960s as a school student, obtained a qualification in design and spoke fluent English. When asked about job opportunities, his perception was that working in Chinese catering was the only way of getting a stable full-time job.

Marcus: What else can you do if not catering? Unless you have a specialty and also you have the contact to get into other areas. If I study in public school, if I worked hard to change my accent it may be easier for me. It's not racial discrimination . . . but to some extent it is a racial discrimination. And they have a misconception.

Author: Doesn't your design qualification help?

Marcus: Design is not a stable job.

Marcus thought that his accent put him at a disadvantage in the job market. He said if he had studied, 'at a royal boarding school', he might be able to embody the 'right' accent, 'I can imitate the accent. But if I have to pretend 100 per cent it will be a headache. I can imitate the accent, the grammar, the tone. But it's difficult. It's not mother tongue for me.'

Accent as a visible sign of ethnic difference was deemed by Marcus to be a barrier. He felt judged and excluded by his accent. It is interesting to note that to be 'socially included', in Marcus' view, one had to speak the 'right' accent, which was Received Pronunciation, an accent associated with the highest social class.

How have the chances of getting Chinese people into the mainstream UK market changed over the years? In a study published in 1999, Pang found an emerging trend of bimodal distribution in which young Chinese adults worked in professions/white collar jobs or were concentrated in the Chinese catering business. However, in research that compared data from the 1991 and 2001 censuses, Chinese people with similar qualifications as White Britons were found to have significantly lower comparative rates of employment (Simpson *et al.*, 2006). Marcus' view that catering still offered the best chances of employment for Chinese people even if they were second generation was rooted in his experience of the substantial barriers to equal employment faced by Chinese people in the UK.

As documented by many studies, participants described working conditions in Chinese restaurants as exploitative (e.g. Baxter, 1988; Kagan *et al.*, 2011). All those participants who had worked in catering said mental health problems were common among the employees of Chinese restaurants. Lai-Ming and Feng had come to the UK in the 1960s and 2000s respectively. Their narratives suggested that the harsh working conditions in the Chinese catering business had remained more or less the same over the years. Lai-Ming described the working conditions in Chinese restaurants during late 1960s and 1970s. He pinpointed the working conditions at the restaurant he was employed in as the reason for his breakdown. He said, 'I worked like a dog. Then I got this mental illness'. He commented on the long working hours common in the Chinese catering business.

> The restaurant was supposed to close at 12am but the boss still let people in at 12:15am. We had so much work to do that when we finally slept it was 2pm. Right after you wake up the next morning you start working. You carry on this pattern for several months . . . Everyone gets crazy. It's difficult not to get crazy if you work like this. For 2 or 3 years, I had to work full weekends too. When other people were happy doing their own stuff at weekend, I had to work like a dog. I did not know how I went through the time at that time.

The cost of running a competitive restaurant business was borne by using every ounce of labour power and expecting workers to do any task required. 'You have to wake up early, clean the toilets, tackle the left over and food residue. Consider yourself lucky if they let you sit in the counter to be cashier.'

A restaurant is a hierarchical workplace with waiters at a low rank.

> As a waiter you are at the receiving end of other people's tempers. Many got nervous breakdown being a waiter. I am not the only one . . . People you work with . . . People in the kitchen shout at you. The boss shouts at you. The customers shout at you.

Lai-Ming said the hard work at the restaurant led to his mental ill health and that it was a widespread phenomenon.

> It's hard work. Won't you get fatigue from working like this? It's a reason why people have nervous breakdowns. It's one factor. A latent factor. Breakdown does not happen suddenly. The mental illness has been latent for a while. When it's time to manifest, it will manifest. You will know. If people around you notice and take you to doctors, you will be fine. If you and people around you ignore it, then it will deteriorate.

Other participant's narratives showed that the working conditions had not improved over time. Feng lived in the restaurant where he worked in the kitchen, ten or more hours a day, six days a week. Looking back, he thought many people working in restaurants, like him, were not 'normal', because 'If the businesses are good, the bosses are ok. But if the business is bad, the boss will lose temper and shout at you'.

Both Lai-Ming and Feng did not mention any strategies for coping with the pressure from the boss or dealing with customers' demands. They seemed to put up with the working conditions, which, when looking back, they said had precipitated breakdowns, and led them leaving their jobs.

As Marcus observed, even though many people showed signs of mental health problems, it was not a topic that workers would talk openly about. Resignation seemed to be the only coping strategies that workers felt able to utilise.

> First, I don't have relatives here. I don't have much entertainment. I am not the kind of people who are calculative trying to better themselves. I just kept working. In terms of work, it did not go well for me. So these all accumulated.

Lack of social support was one reason that led to the deterioration of mental health in the midst of a hard working life. As Chau and Yu (2001) argue, Chinese people in the UK experience a 'double social exclusion'. They are excluded from mainstream society, as well as from other members of Chinese communities. Those with family support, as Lai-Ming mentioned, might be able to spot, in his words, 'abnormal behavior' in the worker. However, a family strategy such as taking a worker to see a doctor is a personalised way of dealing with what is a widespread labour problem. In other words, workers are left to develop individual rather than collective strategies in the face of a persistent structural problem.

Questions arise as to why it is so difficult for workers to retain autonomy and assert any bargaining power in the Chinese catering business and why poor working conditions are accepted as the 'norm' for low-skilled Chinese workers. Kagan *et al.* argue that the Chinese catering business in the UK was akin to a 'self-sustaining micro-economy' (2011: 7). On the surface, it seems that low-skilled workers, especially those without English language skills, benefit from this source of work in what is a relatively 'closed' ethnic business. However, they note that workers collude with their exploitation at work not as a choice, but because of a lack of alternatives.

This suggests that the opportunity structure for would-be or existing Chinese migrants to expand their capability through migrating to the UK is actually preconditioned by the difficulties they have in breaking into the mainstream UK labour market. Putting up with poor working conditions or accepting them as the 'norm' can be understood as an adaptive preference. Kagan *et al.* (2011) highlight how the most vulnerable are prone to exploitation. For example, undocumented migrants like Feng, who had to repay the debt he owed the 'snakehead' (the gang that smuggled him to the UK), had difficulty avoiding exploitative work conditions. During the time of economic recession, the working conditions in the catering business were found to have worsened (Wu *et al.*, 2010).

What Marcus and other participants saw as a relatively secure source of work opportunities for Chinese people, seemed to require the sacrifice of mental well-being. For Lai-Ming and Feng, working conditions in the catering business was what they had to 'recover from'. Both of them, even when they passed the crisis stage, still had to cope with symptoms that made it difficult for them to work, whatever the conditions. Chapter 5 provides an account of how cautious they were about going back to work in Chinese restaurants.

Apart from the impact on the workers themselves, the poor working conditions in Chinese catering had a knock-on effect on the families of the workers. Bai-Xin's husband was beaten up while working in a restaurant for 'moving too slow' and 'getting in the way'. The violence resulted in brain damage and left him unable to work again. He then suffered from serious mental illness and Bai-Xin became his carer. When her considerable caring duties became too stressful for her she fell ill too.

Shun-Tien found the people in the restaurant she worked in treated her well. But the long working hours took a toll on her relationship with her then teenage son. Being the sole earner in the household after her husband died, she did not have time to be with her son who was at that time still grieving for the loss of his father. As a result Shun-Tien's relationship with her son suffered and he became distant.

Overseas brides

The narratives of participants who were overseas brides reflected the ways in which transnational marriage could impact on the capabilities development of women. The overseas brides in this study came from a lower-class background and had limited agency in the arrangements for their marriages in the UK. Arranged marriage abroad was used by Chinese families of lower-class backgrounds to improve their daughters' lives. It was also a source for Chinese men in the UK, especially those come from the lower class, to find future wives. A-Bao, Bai-Xin, Nin-Jin, Pun-Yi, Tang-Yung and Wu-Wei were all in their twenties when they married Chinese migrants in the UK. They married over a period starting in the late 1970s and ending in the 1990s. Many did not actively seek to marry abroad, but met their future husbands through parental arrangements.

Bai-Xin recalled that she was 'passive and indifferent' about her parents' decision to marry her in the UK. Married at a relatively young age, Nin-Jin did not feel that she could object to her parents' decision. It could be argued that choosing to follow her parents' arrangement came out of a sense of filial piety (Salaff, 1981). Nonetheless, Nin-Jin suffered from her compliance later when she found migration was not what she really wanted. She had lived in the UK for 30 years at the time of her interview, and said she still felt homesick. She thought that not getting used to life in the UK had contributed to her becoming ill and being prescribed antipsychotics on a long-term basis.

Nin-Jin: May be I got a lot of stress because I dislike living in a foreign country. I like to stay in Hong Kong. It was my family who wanted me to get married here. It wasn't what I wanted. I don't know if it was because of this that I was very unhappy. Also I was alone.

Author: You haven't got family members or relatives other than in-laws here?

Nin-Jin: No. Things were suppressed inside my heart for a long time. I think it had a huge impact on me.

Their parents often had the impression that marrying abroad meant that their daughter would have a better life. However, this was not necessarily the case and if overseas brides found that they had grievances and dissatisfactions they found it difficult to share these with their parents.

They were also expected to fulfill the expectations of their in-laws to help in family catering businesses, have children and provide care for the wider family. For a long time Nin-Jin's social interaction had been restricted to her in laws and their takeaway business. Because of their lack of English language skills, these participants had restricted social networks from which they could seek help.

'Marrying up' was not necessarily perceived as a blessing by these participants. Wu-Wei's low self-esteem and low sense of security was a narrative of hidden injuries of class and gender that constituted the theme of what she needed to recover from. She met her husband through her family's arrangement and they did not fall in love with each other. Coming from a poor family and without higher education qualifications, she worried that people in her hometown would gossip about her, saying she married for money as her husband was a university graduate and her in-laws were richer than her family. Her low self-esteem also stemmed from being sexually assaulted by a relative when she was young. The effect of this trauma only came to light when she underwent counselling many years after several relapses in the UK. The aftermath of the assault became apparent when she got married and started to have sexual relations with her husband.

> I remember that I gave my first night to my husband on the wedding. People suspected that I wasn't a virgin. This irritated me. I told myself I would give my first night to my husband. Now looking back maybe it's more than the gossip. Before that I was worried that I wasn't a virgin. Because when I was young . . . this is something I didn't tell people for a long time. It was only the last time that I was ill and it came back to me like a volcano. I was sexually assaulted by an uncle in my hometown. I was so scared and dared not tell people about it.

Wu-Wei started to feel the weight of social class hierarchy, compounded by the stress of migration and the occupation of an ethnicised gender role inside the family. She thought of committing suicide when she first came to the UK. Her adjustment problems were rooted in cultural and class differences. She said that sometimes she told her husband that he should have married someone 'better'. 'I am the least educated person in the house. I didn't graduate from the school. I knew nothing when I came here. Just crying.'

She was not used to living with her in-law's family. Her mother-in-law would lecture her about 'Chinese traditions'.

> Maybe when I first came here, I didn't do things in the way they wanted. I wanted to learn a lot of things. I had the self-confidence to learn a lot of things. I wanted to rely on myself instead of other people. Maybe I wanted

to live away from them. My mother-in-law gave me a lot of pressure. She wanted me to live with them until they died, take care of them. In my heart I wanted to live with them too. I struggled. I wanted a home of my own, instead of coming home being shouted at. When I got home I had to rush through my meal and then do things for them, worrying that they would shout at me. I kept crying. I blamed myself for not doing enough. I always condemned myself. I know my mother-in-law is good to me.

The trap she felt was further complicated by the financial support her in-laws gave her parents in China. 'My parents would send me letters telling me to listen and pay respect to the in-laws, because they were merciful to us, not only for bringing me here to UK but also helping my family in China.'

Wu-Wei's worst fear was not being able to survive in the UK if her husband abandoned her because of her low educational level and English skills. She longed to be self-reliant and independent. In Chapter 5, Wu-Wei's development of self-worth and economic independence are described as she began to recover from the hidden injuries of 'marrying up'.

Wu-Wei's worry about being abandoned could be interpreted by a cognitive behaviourist as a 'maladaptive thought' resulting from childhood trauma (e.g. Beck, 1976). But worrying about losing the support of a husband also has a structural basis. Marriage as a guarantee of a secure future for overseas brides might not be delivered in real life. Both Nin-Jin's and Shun-Tien's husbands died and they had to raise their children by themselves. Pun-Yi took her children to a women's refuge after her husband beat her. Tang-Yung's mother introduced her to her ex-husband. But when she arrived in the UK she found out her husband was already married. By then she was already heavily pregnant. And life was very different to what she had anticipated before migrating. Deciding that having to live with his first wife would be mental torture, she sought help from the local authority to move away from her husband as she had no money. After a short stay in a refugee hostel, she was allocated a council house. With a roof over her head, she worked, saved up to buy furniture and started a new chapter in her life. However, the area she lived in was far from safe. Her house was burgled and she lost everything overnight. This was a huge blow and Tang-Yung lost hope in her future in the UK.

Being cheated by her husband and then burgled when she was finding her feet again, made her feel trapped. She went back to mainland China. However, when she returned home, she said that her mother 'tricked' her into going to a psychiatric hospital. She lost trust in her family and returned to the UK. On her return she sought help from a Chinese community centre, applied for welfare benefits and started seeing doctors in the UK. Although she was on a regular medication injection, she did not think she was mentally ill. She said she was unhappy and had financial problems because of the vicious cycle of compulsive shopping and debt that she was in. This was how Tang-Yung described her recovery journey: 'Whenever I saw some light, there would be things that brought me down again'.

Caring work: informal carers

Some women participants described the demanding care work they did as a major factor contributing to their mental ill health and distress. The pattern of caring work falling disproportionately on women in a family household is not exclusive to the Chinese culture. The subordination of women in the domestic sphere and their caring work has been identified as a manifestation of capitalism and patriarchy in Western countries (Dalley, 1988). However, the ethnic ideology of 'the traditional Chinese way of doing things' is often appropriated as a disciplining force to justify keeping women in the domestic sphere. In situations where full-time caring for adults and children at home is necessary, the lack of public caring services means that the family has to resort to private strategies based on familism. The narratives of Abao and Bai-Xin revealed how the heavy burdens of care they carried led both of them to breaking point.

When Abao first met her husband, her in-laws hid from her that her husband had severe learning difficulties and required full-time attention and care. She had agreed to a marriage in the UK as her married sister lived there and wanted her company. She only met her husband a few times before they married and she thought he was quiet. After their marriage she realised her husband required a lot of care and attention from her. He did not recognise street signs or distinguish day from night. She had to take care of the husband as well as three children. Her husband wanted to prove that he could manage things but he could not express himself. His temper got worse as he got older. One day he left home after a row. It was only then that her in-laws told her about his learning difficulties and his past history of attempting suicide.

This incident made her decide to try to bottle up her own emotions in order not to trigger his temper again. Her relationship with her in-laws was tense. They wanted her to have a son to maintain their lineage. They also suspected her of hiding the benefits due to her husband and children. She was offered a job but she said her mother-in-law would not let her take it as she was worried that Abao would leave her husband if she met other people. Gradually Abao's physical and mental health deteriorated.

Bai-Xin said that she did not ask for a high quality of life when she got married. Her focus was on her husband and children and she was reluctant to spend money on herself. The family's aim was to save enough money for a house. When her third daughter was about 4 months old, her husband was beaten up in the restaurant he worked in. His head injury resulted in a persistent mental health problem. This happened at a time when she felt unwell after giving birth to her daughter. Her husband lost his ability to work, they had to sell their house and apply for benefits. It was getting difficult to live with her husband and when he was sectioned she lost control of herself. She cried all the time, felt frightened, and sometimes did not know who she was. She frantically phoned her friends to the point where she risked losing them. Although she was her husband's main carer and went with him to the psychiatrist, her own mental health condition went unnoticed by the doctor.

Abao's and Bai-Xin's husbands relied heavily on them. They did not like to go out and they did not want Abao and Bai-Xin to go out without them. Abao and Bai-Xin planned their lives around their husbands. Although they were both eager to learn English in order improve their communications in daily life, and enjoyed the few English lessons they managed to attend, the attention their husbands demanded from them made it difficult for them to continue. Before they sought help, they felt that they had to sacrifice their well-being for the family. As Abao put it, 'Sometimes when I think of taking care of myself, I feel that it means neglecting the family'.

For informal carers like Abao and Bai-Xin, what they had to recover from was a caring regime built on the sacrifice of their capabilities.

Childbirth

Several women participants pointed to childbirth as one of the causes, if not the sole cause, of their mental distress. Entering parenthood was a big turning point in the lives of several participants (see, for example, Feng's narrative about becoming a father outlined earlier). However, women faced additional challenges linked to bodily changes and birth risks. Poor health and post-natal depression was not just about the hormonal changes. The lack of support systems these participants experienced after childbirth together with the demands of caring for a newborn baby could easily make too great a demand on their coping capacities.

Abao, Bai-Xin and Nin-Jin recalled that they started feeling unwell after giving birth. However, they did not seek help when they started to experience distress and so lost the opportunity of accessing support through midwives' visits. Bai-Xin felt that her physical health weakened after giving birth to her third daughter. She became sensitive to heat and felt 'spaced out' for no reason. In retrospect she recalled that she did not give herself enough space to 'do the month', i.e. rest after childbirth because of the stress of taking care of her other children. 'Doing the month' is a cultural practice in Chinese culture that requires women to stay indoors to recover from childbirth (Holroyd *et al.*, 1997). It is beyond the scope of this study to discuss this cultural practice and the different ways Chinese women perceive it. However, it is noteworthy that Bai-Xin in mentioning it indicated that she had wanted support rooted in traditional Chinese medical concepts of 'cold' and 'heat' and yin and yang, in dealing with her difficulties.

Bai-Xin experienced her poor health as a pressure. She did not tell the midwives who visited her how she was feeling. She said this was because she did not know how to describe her feeling of being 'spaced out' in English.

> When I looked in the mirror, I couldn't recognise myself. I asked myself who was the person in the mirror. I did not recognise the person I saw in the mirror. When I went outside, I felt like I was drunk. I felt my head was hot and swollen. I felt like I had changed. I felt sad when communicating with people.

At that time, she did not consider that the distress she was experiencing was an illness and that she could seek help for from the midwife, 'At that time I didn't feel that I was a patient. I felt that I was crazy. If I realised that I was ill . . . I felt ill, but I could not pinpoint where and how I felt ill'.

The midwife did not pick up her distress. Bai-Xin suggested that this was because she had had no problems during labour. While she could not articulate what was wrong, she knew it was totally different to how she felt after the births of her first two children. She felt that her 'whole person' had changed but she did not tell her in-laws or friends about it, as she thought it was something she had to put up with as an overseas bride.

> When I came from China to here, to my husband . . . how did I feel that time . . . giving birth to children, bringing them up, buying a house, husband working, taking care of the household . . . I didn't think of other things. There are ups and downs, but I didn't consider it as hardship. I didn't ask for a high quality of life. I didn't ask for pretty clothes. What I focused on was husband working and us saving for a house. I didn't spend money on other things. I was reluctant to spend money to make myself happy. I didn't buy anything. The money my husband brought home was all saved up for buying a house.
>
> I only realised later on that I was stupid. Life for myself shouldn't be like this. If a person carries on like this for a whole life, it will be a meaningless life.

It is quite common in Chinese societies that parents, especially mothers, take care of their daughters after they give birth. Bai-Xin did not have the choice to give birth in her home country where she might have received more support from her parents.

In contrast, Carol chose to give birth to her first child in Hong Kong, where she felt more at ease and had parental support. Carol recalled that she showed signs of what she now knew was post-natal depression, right after her son was born. However, she was not aware of what it was at the time. She had attended a seminar organised by the hospital in Hong Kong during her pregnancy. A nurse had mentioned post-natal depression at the seminar, but had not talked about symptoms or what it felt like. When Carol 'did the month' in Hong Kong, she had support from her parents, but she did not think she had had enough rest as she had to keep waking up to feed the baby. Many friends and relatives visited her and the baby, and this became a source of stress for Carol as it took up the time she needed to recover from sleep deprivation. Not long after the birth her husband flew back to his job in the UK, so he was no longer there to support her.

Carol's mother flew back with her to the UK after she 'did the month'. However her support was time limited as 6 months is the longest period her mother could stay with a Hong Kong passport. Carol was sectioned, under the Mental Health Act with post-natal depression shortly after her return to the UK. When she was in the early stages of her recovery there was little support for her and the baby. As Carol's narrative shows (see more in Chapter 5), this meant that she struggled to keep up her caring work for her household and child. Carol's socio-economic position was good compared to other participants, but this had limited effect in compensating for her lack of social networks in the UK.

These participant's narratives suggest that the NHS midwives who visited them focused on the practicalities of caring for newborn babies. Carol observed that they seemed to put more emphasis on teaching her to take care of the baby, rather than her own well-being. However, the healthy development of a newborn baby is premised on the well-being of the mother. A mother cannot use her nurturing skills in practice if she is in mental distress. What seems to be lacking in the midwifery service is mental health training.

The participants' narratives indicated that they decided to put up with the discomforts they experienced rather than talk about them with their midwives. Bai-Xin illustrated how some overseas brides had normalised the hardship of their lives in the UK by putting their husband's and family's needs before their own. Adapting to a life centered on the family gave them an anchor or life goal in a new country, but this came at the cost of putting their own needs on hold and neglecting their own well-being.

Even though Nin-Jin knew that her recovery after giving birth to her third daughter was more difficult than with her previous births, she thought that the mental distress she experienced had to be endured. This adaptive preference meant that these overseas brides lowered their expectations of personal well-being and did not seek help in until they reached crisis point.

Aging and isolation

Aging and isolation was another factor mentioned by participations who had been overseas brides. They often referred to their children as being their 'hope', their achievement and a source of consolation. However, for some this was far from the case. When Shun-Tien migrated to the UK with her husband and their son, she only met other people through her husband. When her husband died not long after they settled in the UK, her son was about 10 years old. Shun-Tien decided to stay in the UK for her son's sake. Her son, who had adored his father, did not cope very well with his death and started to become distanced from her. Although she received financial support from the local authority, she had to work to make ends meet. She had no time to talk with her son and dealt with her own grief and loneliness with work and sleeping pills. Her relations with her son deteriorated and one day she found he had stolen money from her.

At the time of the interview Shun-Tien was estranged from her only family member in the UK. She was lonely, but preferred to keep her independence instead of going to live in a home for the elderly. She worried about gossips and although she was invited by the Chinese community centre to join in the activities for older people she seldom attended. Worrying about people gossiping reflects not only her small social network, it also related to the difficulties faced in 'breaking into' a close-knit group. So Shun-Tien preferred to be a bystander at the centre. 'When I go there I only chat with Ms Chan (staff). When I see them playing mahjog and doing exercises, I feel happy for them. Seeing people happy makes me feel happy too'.

In-Lei also experienced loneliness. She considered isolation as the cause of her distress. She lived in a housing association flat some way from the city where her grown up daughter lived. She did not trust people easily and attributed this to her experience of 'backstabbing' colleagues when she had worked in mainland China. She thought her low self-esteem was a result of not being able to work in the UK and not having a son (according to ideology in Chinese cultures, particularly in rural areas, giving birth to a son means continuity of the 'ancestral lineage' and is considered an achievement or a sense of 'duty' fulfilled. A woman's failure to have a son can be experienced as a failure in life). In-Lei tried working for a Chinese employer but left when she found that he did not earn his money honestly and became worried that she would be caught. She had taken several English classes in the UK. However, her limited contact with other people meant that she had no one to practice her English with. She thought her English was not good enough to find an 'English job'.

Now in her sixties, In-Lei said she 'dared not to hope' as she lived in a host country and had heart problems. She worried about living on her own in case she had a heart attack. She found having to deal with household maintenance problems difficult and stressful. When she encountered a bureaucratic obstacle, she took it personally and it reinforced her distrust of others. Her distrust of others and her worry about retaliation made her wary about using health and social care services. How to build trust and connectedness was a recovery theme for her, as well as for other older participants.

Conclusions

This chapter critically considered and analysed the social conditions that contributed to participants' mental ill health. The key argument is that the diminishment of mental well-being is often a result of capabilities deprivation related to the intersectional inequalities of positionality. On an individual level, capabilities deprivation becomes a theme of what to recover from, into long-term recovery journeys. Recovery involves addressing the capabilities deprivation that rendered service users vulnerable in the first place. Using the Capabilities Approach as a heuristic device in this research, I have teased out various vulnerable factors for Chinese people in the UK. Agency, as a central tenet of the Capabilities Approach and the constitutive element of an individual's capabilities set, is important to mental health well-being. As the data reveals, citizenship, working conditions and caring work can place limitations on an individual's agency and so adversely affect mental well-being. This chapter provides a baseline from which to evaluate the recovery journey of the participants in subsequent chapters. It poses the question of whether mental health problems can be traced to capabilities deprivations associated with individuals' social locations, and how these capabilities develop along their recovery journeys.

The data in this chapter showed how class, gender and ethnicity intersected in ways that resulted in the expansion or contraction of exercisable opportunities in the capabilities of individuals. Looking at life stages spanning from young adult to old age, and examining the institutions of citizenship, education, labour market, marriage and family, the narratives of the participants provided insights into what was needed for recovery at macro and collective levels. As members of an ethnic minority in the UK, the participants' predicaments also reflected class and gender inequalities. Their biographies as well as the processes leading to their distress and ill health were clearly gendered. Moreover, the intersection of class, gender and ethnicity has a transnational dimension. For example, the situation of overseas brides results from the social location of Chinese men in the UK, lower class women in mainland China as well as the global North–South divide in which people from less developed countries seek better life chances in more developed countries.

Deep contextualisation of recovery journeys through the lens of local and transnational social hierarchies is important for two reasons. First, on an individual level it gives a fuller picture of the needs, as well as the capabilities, of the service users. Individuals are not, first and foremost, Chinese or a service user. It also provides for the development of holistic person-centered care, an understanding of the struggles and life challenges service users face due to interweaving structural barriers based on class, gender and aging, which negatively impact on their mental well-being. Second, an individual's exercisable opportunities are predicated on possibilities in the social structure. This means that individual recovery cannot be separated from changes required at a sociostructural level. This indicates a need to develop collective capabilities utilising a community development approach (Ibrahim, 2006). The data generated by the narratives of informal carers is illustrative here. It highlights a need to have environmental conversion factors in the form of public care and subsidies instead of leaving caring work to be privately dealt with, which results in diminishing the capabilities of the carer as well as the cared for.

While the process leading to mental ill health is a process of capabilities loss or deprivation, seeking and receiving help and care should be about halting the diminishment of capabilities, developing deprived capabilities and/or redeveloping lost capabilities. This brings us to the next chapter, which explores participants' pathways to care and their experiences of becoming a psychiatric patient. The features of psychiatry are examined together with participants' experiences, in order to discover whether capabilities essential to mental health were developed during the process.

4 Becoming a psychiatric patient

Introduction

This chapter explores how participants experienced the pathologisation and medicalisation processes of mental distress and reflects on whether these processes were capability enhancing or diminishing. Chapter 3 considered the social conditions that contributed to the deterioration of the mental health of the participants and led to a period of 'shipwreck', a metaphor used in the Tidal Model for acute mental health crisis or breakdown (Barker and Buchanan-Barker, 2005). This chapter sheds light on participants' pathways to care and their experiences of becoming psychiatric patients. It considers the diagnostic process, the different treatments received and hospitalisation. It raises a number of issues including the ways that processes enabled or hindered the redevelopment of mental well-being capability. It looks at how the agency of participants was respected, nurtured or violated, as well as providing an account of the options the participants were presented with during medical encounters.

The process leading to mental ill health is conceptualised as a process of capabilities loss or deprivation. In contrast, seeking and receiving help and care is considered as a process that has the potential of halting the diminishment of capabilities, developing the deprived capabilities and/or redeveloping the capabilities lost. This chapter gives particular consideration to whether the experience of being a member of an ethnic minority places individuals at a disadvantage when using the UK mental health system. A focus on the context of psychiatric power is also maintained in order to shed light on whether participants benefitted from different interventions in redeveloping their mental well-being and daily functioning, as well as whether sanism and psychiatric power started to shape participants' biographies during the process of pathologisation and medicalisation. The way that power inequalities intersect is analysed at two levels. First, the way that gender, class and other factors contribute to the diversity of experience within Chinese communities. Second, how pathologisation and medicalisation intersect with ethnicity and other structural factors in shaping service users' experiences of psychiatry.

Participants' experience of psychiatry was located in the UK, Hong Kong and mainland China. Nine out of the 22 participants had used mental health services in their home countries before or after coming to the UK. The psychiatric system in Hong Kong follows the UK system closely (Hong Kong was a UK colony from 1841 to 1997). In contrast, mainland China has its own diagnostic manual, the *Chinese Classification of Mental Disorders* (CCMD; Chinese Society of Psychiatry, 2001). Its psychiatric system is dominated by the bio-medical model and has powers to compulsorily detain people in hospital as in the UK and Hong Kong. There are of course differences in terms of the configuration of mental health services and the degrees of patients' rights in different countries. For example, in the UK, straightjacket and physical constraints are banned in institutions and service configurations reflect a process of deinstitutionalisation that started in the last quarter of the twentieth century. Physical restraints are still used in mainland China and Hong Kong. It is not within the scope of this research to compare and discuss the three different systems. In this chapter the place in which a participants' experience took place is named when context is needed to make sense of the narrative.

This chapter is in three sections. The first section considers the process of entering the medical encounter and the role of language capability in this process. The next section goes on to look at participants' experiences in the various stages of medicalisation: receiving a diagnosis, treatments and interventions, and hospitalisation. The final section discusses in what ways medicalisation can be considered as an 'incomplete' project of colonisation of a lifeworld by using the detailed narrative of one participant (Habermas, 1987; Scambler, 2002; Barker, 2003), and how this incomplete project related to that person's agency.

Pathways to care: structure and process

Pathways to health care are part of a social process shaped by social and cultural factors (Armstrong, 1994; Morgan *et al.*, 2004). Focusing on aspects of the 'opportunities' dimension and the 'process' dimension as delineated in the Capabilities Approach, the structure of the health care system in respect to its available services can be scrutinised as to whether it is capability enhancing and respects agency.

Utilisation of plural medical models

Some participants had seen traditional Chinese medicine practitioners in mainland China, Hong Kong and the UK. It was a way to maximise their health care resources especially when the causes or the nature of the distress and ill health was unclear. It was often used, alongside accessing GPs, when participants were uncertain as to whether their distress was a mental health problem, especially when it was experienced as physical illness.

Marcus's mental ill health started with severe headaches. He first went to his GP, who, he said, had exhausted all the possible tests but still couldn't pinpoint what was wrong with him. The Chinese medicine prescribed cleared his headache, but his mental state continued to deteriorate. Similarly, out of pragmatism,

Zoie started using Chinese medicine for her depression in Hong Kong when she found her prescribed antidepressant was not very helpful. However, as Chinese medical practitioners are predominately located in private practices in the UK, she was deterred from using Chinese medicine there because of the expense. Jerry's parents took him to see a Chinese medical practitioner in the UK when he started experiencing mental distress. He did not stay with the practitioner as he preferred the speed of Western medicine compared to Chinese medicine. Abao shared this view and did not go to see a Chinese practitioner when she was desperate for a doctor to cure her severe abdominal pain. However, after a series of check-ups with NHS consultants, she eventually found relief for her pain after treatment in a hospital in mainland China that combined Western and Chinese medicine methods.

Abao's pathway to care was a long process of working out whether her somatisation of depression (Kleinman, 1977), was a physical illness or not. Utilisation of plural medical models as well as transnational usage of health care systems seemed to facilitate the process and helped Abao relieve her pain and discomfort. When she first sought help for her pain Abao was diagnosed as depressed by her GP due to her heavy caring responsibilities. She was prescribed tranquillisers, but when her intestinal pain persisted she kept going to the GP for check-ups, to the point when she thought the GP was reluctant to see her. She then went to see a Chinese-speaking private Western medicine doctor, who referred her for more hospital tests, including a CT scan and gynecological tests. Nothing was found and her pain persisted. The hospital consultant said her pain was a somatic symptom of depression. The turning point came when the consultant asked her if she had thought of going back to China for treatment, as they had exhausted what they could do for her in the UK. However, she was worried that no one would take care of her daughters and husband while she was away. She was also worried that if the NHS knew that she had had medical care outside the UK she would lose 'her place' in the NHS. The consultant reassured her that this would not happen and arranged to see her when she came back from China. Eventually she went to a hospital in mainland China that combined Western and Chinese medicine treatments. She was diagnosed as having an inflammatory bowel disease. She underwent hydrotherapy and took a combination of Chinese herbal medicines as well as antidepressants. Her pain was finally relieved.

Several points emerge from Abao's experience in terms of capability enhancement. First, she seemed to encounter a barrier at the GPs. Her narrative raised the question of whether she had experienced 'diagnostic overshadowing' with the GP who did not refer her on for a specialist checkup. 'Diagnostic overshadowing', as Thornicroft *et al.* argue, is commonly found in general health care settings (2007: 113). It occurs when practitioners mistakenly assume physical illness signs and symptoms are linked to a concurrent mental illness diagnosis. Service users want to recover from both their physical and mental distress. Abao did not deny she had depression. But she did not accept that it was the reason for the abdominal pain. The treatment for depression she received in the UK did not relieve her abdominal pain. Abao might also have experienced a disadvantage as a result of not being able to speak fluent English, as it seems that she only managed to access further testing after seeing a Chinese-speaking practitioner. In the lengthy and draining process of finding out what is the wrong and what the right treatment is, enabling service users to access different services and treatments is important. It is possible that Abao's stomach pain was a sign of mental distress and the accumulated distress resulted in the physical manifestation of a tumor that happened much later, after rounds of check-ups by the consultant in specialist care in the UK. It could also be that a month's break from her intensive work caring for her family allowed her to relax and rejuvenate.

It is not in the scope of this book to discuss the strength and weakness of different medical models. However, a consultants' facilitation of the use of other medical models as well as health care in other countries enabled Abao to get the right treatments. What the consultant did was to maintain Abao's help-seeking capability in terms of respecting her agency. Instead of insisting that her physical pain was solely a somatic symptom of depression, she was encouraged to use other health care systems without burning her bridges in relation to accessing the UK health system.

Transnational usage of health care systems

Like Abao, other participants who broke down in the UK had used health care systems in mainland China and Hong Kong at their crisis point. For some too, this counterweighed the barriers they might have experienced as members of an ethnic minority in a hospital setting.

When Lai-Ming was admitted to a UK psychiatric hospital, the doctor arranged for him to be treated in a public psychiatric hospital in Hong Kong, thinking that it would be best for him to be treated in his home country where he might feel more at ease in a familiar cultural environment. Family members accompanied him to Hong Kong and visited him when he was hospitalised. The capabilities deprivation that ethnic minority members face can be addressed by transnational usage of health care in their home country, as well as in the UK. However, such arrangements remain a privilege for those who can afford to travel and have a support system they can draw on in their home country. It cannot be assumed that all Chinese people in the UK have the resources needed to access transnational health care systems.

Several participants' narratives illustrated that pathways to health care systems in their home country was not always a positive experience. For some it was experienced as capability diminishing. Marcus and Wu-Wei were admitted to a hospital through emergency services in Hong Kong when they planned to go to mainland China. For Tang-Yung, it was a negative pathway, involving coercion that adversely affected her willingness to engage with mental health services (Morgan *et al.*, 2004). She said that she was tricked by her family and compulsorily admitted to a psychiatric hospital during her visit back home to mainland

China. Not only did she continue to find it difficult to develop trust in mental health services, she also lost trust in her family in mainland China.

Language capability, interpretation services and assertiveness in exercising agency in medical encounters

In terms of using UK health care services, language capability emerged as an important condition for exercising agency during medical encounters. Clinicians cannot 'validate' a psychiatric diagnosis using physical tests but rely heavily on service users' as well as carers and observations. A service user's ability to express and articulate their distress is important to help clinicians clarify the nature of the problems they face as well as understanding the crisis they are experiencing. For Chinese service users who have limited English language skills, competent interpretation is important in making sure they are not deprived of their language capability.

Not all the participants were aware that they could request an interpretation service when using the NHS. For example, In-Lei had lived in the UK for over 10 years but it was only recently that she and her daughter, who could speak English, learnt that the NHS could provide interpreters. Some participants relied on family members, partners or children as interpreters. This meant they could only arrange medical appointments when family members were available. It could be difficult to arrange a time that was feasible for all parties, especially if the only family member they could rely on was working full-time. Also, it should not be assumed that all participants have family members to rely on for interpretation. In-Lei's daughter lived far away so she relied on friends or neighbours to interpret for her. She paid them for their help. Such informal arrangements were experienced as stressful by In-Lei. She worried that friends talked behind her back if she failed to pay them and she would lose their friendship and help. When she started to use statutory interpreters, her stress about her friends was relieved. Dependence on informal social networks can make an individual vulnerable to manipulation. In-Lei recalled a friend who offered to interpret for her but demanded that she had to hire her exclusively for all the interpretation she needed. In-Lei agreed to this but was let down when the interpreter failed to show up on time, which resulted in her having to cancel her long awaited appointment.

Both Carol and In-Lei found that the quality of interpreters they got from NHS and the community centre was patchy. Once In-Lei was prescribed the wrong medication for an unrelated illness. She only found this out when a Mandarin-speaking pharmacist checked the medicine with her. It was not only that the interpretation she was getting was not carefully done, sentence by sentence, that made her suspicious of its accuracy. The interpreter was Malaysian and although she spoke Cantonese, In-Lei felt that she did not understand the subtle cultural meanings of expressions used in Hong Kong Cantonese. On one occasion Carol thought her interpreter managed to interpret correctly but panicked when Carol broke down in tears during the consultation. Carol found this both irritating and unhelpful. Such bad experiences seem all too common among ethnic minority members, leading to a general lack of confidence in professional interpreters (Fountain and Hicks, 2010).

Worry about gossip was another factor that had stopped some participants from using statutory and Chinese community centre services. Confidentiality was not always treated seriously. Worrying that her privacy would be invaded and she would face discrimination from the Chinese community, Carol preferred to get through medical consultations using her own limited English vocabulary when her husband was not available to interpret for her.

Generally service providers relied on family members or friends to interpret for service users, but there were occasions when family members were not allowed to act as interpreters. Assessment leading to sectioning for compulsory treatment was one example. In these circumstances the statutory interpretation service was used. There was no choice – it was forced upon participants. In Carol's experience, this was very problematic as she sensed that the interpreters did not convey her exact meanings, which, in her view, led to her subsequent compulsory hospitalisation. This was a grievance that Carol carried with her as she moved forward on her recovery journey.

When participants found interpretation arranged by community centres helpful, it was because meticulous sentence-by-sentence interpretation was carried out and service users knew and trusted the interpreters. These interpreters usually had an understanding of mental health issues, as well as the persons they interpreted for.

Pun-Yi said she had developed trust in her interpreter and this enabled her to feel at ease when seeing her doctor. It seems that in such circumstances good interpreters provided more than translation, they mediated the relationship between the service user and the doctor, as an advocate would. However, even in these circumstances, subtle yet important communications that contributed to recovery could be lost. Developing trusting relationships with the professionals is of central importance to long-term mental health service users. At the same time professionals need to get to know the person in order to develop person-centered recovery plans. Making sense of ill health, as well as the recovery journey, was important for service users in regaining control of their lives.

Carol described vividly the feeling of having to converse through an interpreter. She said she felt like a 'hairy crab' (*Da Zha Xie*, a seasonal Chinese food). These crabs are sold with their legs and claws tightly wrapped with hay straws. Carol's imagery conveyed the feeling of being 'tied up' and prevented from expressing and asserting herself. It is a vivid description of the feelings of trapped agency. Carol felt that it was important for her to be able to share her private and inner feelings, so as to build trust with the professionals. But neither by using her limited English, or an interpreter, did she feel able to achieve this trust with her doctor. Conveying her feelings through a third party felt awkward.

> Sometimes for private matters, it is difficult to tell the doctor through the interpreter. I feel like chatting with the interpreter, not the doctor. I think this is the greatest problem we people with mental distress face. It's difficult to build a relationship with the doctor.

Behind these communication problems was the anticipation, by some participants, that they would build a trusting relationship with doctors in which they would seek explanations for the distress and crisis they experienced. However those who had used services long term said that it was difficult to bring up their concerns, because each medical consultation became a routine about 'maintenance' with the clinicians settling into a standard 'script'.

During her interview, Nin-Jin kept asking me questions about why she had mental illness, for example, whether it was inherited from her mother who suffered from neurasthenia, and whether neurasthenia was the same as schizophrenia. Neurasthenia, also known as *shenjing shuairuo*, is not just a diagnosis that was once commonly used in China (Lee and Kleinman, 2007). It was also used in Western medicine until it was replaced by depressive and anxiety disorder as a diagnostic category (Taylor, 2001). Although Nin-Jin had been a long-term service user, it occurred to me that there were many questions that seemed to be important to her, which she had not asked. It was a language problem, Nin-Jin said, that prevented her from asking the questions she wanted to ask even though she was accompanied by an interpreter. Nin-Jin's unspoken concern was crucial to her recovery in terms of self-understanding and making sense of the crisis she had experienced. Participants' narratives suggested that such concerns were not often addressed in medical encounters and the problem went beyond whether the professional was sympathetic. Nin-Jin considered medical professionals 'clever and experienced', and thought they were able to help her. It seemed that assertiveness was required on the part of participants to bring up issues outside of the professionally defined script of the medical encounter. This was difficult because these encounters were usually defined by the professionals, and this balance of power needed to change if service users were to take the driving seat in their recovery journeys.

While the above experiences illustrated the barriers faced by migrants with limited knowledge of the English language, it also shows how seeking medical help for mental and psychological distress is one that requires service users to articulate and express their suffering. Participants were often in a vulnerable state in a medical encounter and having a relationship of trust with clinicians was considered important to them. Language capability was a key factor in building trust as well as understanding a doctor's explanations and talking about their own distress. However, there were other factors that impacted on building a trusting relationship, which will now be discussed.

Receiving a diagnosis

Receiving a psychiatric diagnosis is one of the 'thresholds' of entering into the medicalisation process. As Jutel (2011: 4) puts it,

> The process of diagnosis provides the framework within which medicine operates, punctuates the values that medicine espouses, and underlines the authoritative role of both medicine and the doctor. Diagnosis takes place at

a salient juncture between illness and disease, patient and doctor, complaint and explanation.

Participants' experiences of receiving a diagnosis illustrated the authoritative role of both medicine and the doctor. This was reflected in the prescription of treatments according to the diagnostic decision as well as the role of diagnosis in shaping participants' understanding of the crisis and distress they experienced. In terms of the diagnostic process, its cultural and social dimensions were not just a 'translation' or 'matching' of experiences and feelings in one's lifeworld with the framework of pathologisation. Bradley's (2006: 138) phrase 'the "fuzziness" of diagnosis' describes well the uncertainties of the diagnosis process, the blurred boundaries between mentally 'ill' and 'well', and between different diagnoses found in the accounts of the participants. Table 4.1 shows the varieties of diagnosis received as reported by the participants.

Several participants were not sure about their diagnosis, even though they had received one according to workers in the Chinese community centre and they were on long-term psychiatric medications. For example, a worker told me that Shun-Tien had depression. She was prescribed sleeping pills for more than 10 years and she said she could not sleep without them. However she did not know what her diagnosis was. Tang-Yung had regular injections of a psychiatric drug once every two weeks, but she was not sure what her diagnosis was. She said that the doctor might have told the nurse but not her, in both the hospital in China and the UK. Nin-Jin had been in hospital several times and was on a long-term antipsychotic drug. She suspected her diagnosis was schizophrenia but she was not sure as the doctor only prescribed medication when they met.

Diagnosis has importance for the redevelopment of an individual's mental health capability. Godderis (2011) argued that knowing their official diagnosis can help service users to negotiate for services. Shun-Tien, Nin-Jin and Tang-Yung relied on Chinese community centre workers to access their mental health services. This meant that the task of negotiation for services was taken up by support workers who could interpret. For them, if they did not understand what

Table 4.1 Diagnosis received as reported by participants

- Schizophrenia
- Schizo-affective disorder
- Hebephrenia
- Paranoid schizophrenia
- Delusion
- Bipolar mood disorder
- Post-natal depression
- Depression
- Mixed anxiety and depressive disorder
- Stress and anxiety
- 'Unhappiness'
- Unknown

was going on, even with interpreters present at their medical consultations, they had their support workers to discuss their concerns with.

For Shun-Tien, knowing her diagnosis did not matter as long as her medication helped her sleep and stop 'thinking too much'. Tang-Yung and Nin-Jin found the diagnosis or the pathologising of their distress as mental illness problematic. Tang-Yung did not agree that she was mentally ill in the sense of a biological illness as she felt that her distress was primarily a result of constant setbacks in her life. The problematic of the pathologisation process reflected in the way Nin-Jin kept wondering and pondering what her 'illness' was. As I illustrate later, Nin-Jin not being sure what her diagnosis was could be understood as her feeling that a bio-medical diagnosis was insufficient in helping her to make sense of her condition. How different participants perceived their diagnosis is now explored.

Ambivalence towards diagnosis: users' negotiation with and distance from the label

Ken, Marcus, Wu-Wei and Zoie expressed ambivalence about their diagnoses. Their ambivalence reflected the way the sick role could give service users a sense of relief through legitimising a state of being that felt strange or unfamiliar to them. At the same time this 'sick role' can perpetuate self-stigma for service users, encouraging them to make sense of their experience in terms of 'normalcy' and 'pathology'.

When Zoie was first told that she suffered from depression, she felt relieved that her sudden experience of distressing intrusive suicidal urges was given a name. Ken and Marcus found it useful as they were able to seek help from health services because of their diagnoses. Wu-Wei had had compulsory hospitalisation in Hong Kong and in mainland China, but she did not know what her diagnosis was. She said she had not asked about her condition as she was too ill. Her husband dealt with the hospital issues so she did not know what was going on. She was not informed about her diagnosis before discharge, nor did she come out with an increased understanding of her mental health conditions. She had only been told that she had bipolar disorder in her most recent UK admission. After her discharge she had looked up what bipolar disorder meant on the Internet and discussed the diagnosis with her Chinese-speaking counsellor. Familiarising herself with the diagnosis had meant that she had gradually learnt how to understand her own emotions and how to cope with her highs and lows; knowing her diagnosis also enabled her to manage her condition by being aware of signs that suggested the possibility of relapse.

However, these positive effects of knowing about a diagnosis came with its devastating labelling effects. For some participants, it meant capability diminishment brought about by a loss of significant relationships and self-stigmatisation. Marcus experienced a loss of relationships as his wife divorced him after knowing his diagnosis was 'paranoid schizophrenia'. Wu-Wei read about bipolar disorder in Chinese. She contemplated the term 'manic depression', which has a similar translation in Chinese signifying 'manic' and 'depression', as opposed to the translation of 'bipolar', which signifies 'variation into two polarity'. 'Manic' can mean 'crazy' in Chinese. As Wu-Wei said, 'I read about the term *zaokuangy-iyuzheng*. I was thinking how I would become *zaokuang*. I was really worried that I would go crazy.'

Wu-Wei even went to the doctor and asked if she would become crazy and violent one day. Her doctor reassured her that looking at her history she had a 'good kind' of bipolar. Although Wu-Wei learnt more about her diagnosis and ways to take care of herself, it was not a clear-cut acceptance.

> I think not many Chinese at the beginning would want to admit they have mental illness. Because 'crazy' and 'mad' are vocabulary used to insult people. Also in my hometown, some girls who were said to be 'mad' were being locked up, being used to work for others. So this is what I came into contact [with] in the past. I still would ask myself why I had this illness. I think about life . . . sometimes I accept it, sometimes I don't.

Wu-Wei's ambivalence about mental illness was common among the participants. On the one hand, Wu-Wei knew about how mental illness was stigmatised and the demeaning status of service users in her hometown, and she did not want to identify with them. On the other hand, she agonised over her life, asking why she became 'one of them'.

While Wu-Wei agonised over the highly stigmatising Chinese translation of her diagnosis, some participants were given 'informal labels' instead of one of the official diagnoses in the *Diagnostic and Statistical Manual of Mental Disorders* or the *International Classification of Diseases* as shown in Table 4.1. These informal labels did not mean that their mental health problem were less severe. For example, the doctor told Lai-Ming that his diagnosis was 'stress and anxiety', after he had been hospitalised and his ill health impacted on his job seeking. Informal labels can be understood as a device professionals use to avoid jargon or reduce the stigmatisation of service users. However, Dobransky (2011) has argued that the informal labels used by workers, e.g. 'common' or 'severe', serve the function of social control just as formal labels do. The dichotomy of 'normal' and 'abnormal' ran through Lai-Ming's narrative when he described his medical encounters. One of his symptoms, he said, was 'abnormal behavior'. 'The conversation is not as natural, because we are not normal people. Abnormal, you could say. When you reply to the doctors, they will forgive you saying abnormal things, because you are patients.'

It seems that replacing official labels with less stigmatising ones did not remove the pathologisation and the notion of 'ab/normalcy', which defined Lai-Ming's sense of his mental health crisis and continuing distress. The disciplining effect of 'ab/normalcy' was apparent in his narratives on his job seeking and disability experience (see Chapters 5 and 6 for details).

Diagnosis in the context of power

Apart from the labelling effects of diagnosis discussed above that reflect prejudices in communities, labelling exists within the psychiatric professions. The definition of what is unacceptable behavior, which is then pathologised in psychiatry, is value-laden. Zoie received a diagnosis of borderline personality disorder (BPD) that lasted a week during her hospitalisation in Hong Kong. The experience gave her an acute awareness of the operation of power in psychiatry. Her experience not only revealed the controversy and the 'arbitrariness' of psychiatric diagnosis classification. It also revealed the power relationships between professionals and service users within a Hong Kong hospital setting.

Zoie's diagnosis had been 'mixed anxiety and depressive disorder'. During her hospitalisation, her doctors decided that her diagnosis should be 'borderline personality disorder'. The treatment plan remained mostly unchanged apart from her receiving an additional antipsychotic drug, which was not for treating the new diagnosis but for symptomatic relief. She was also told that psychotherapy for borderline personality disorder would last longer than that usually given for depression. For Zoie the treatment plan did not change much from what she expected. Being severely depressed and feeling hopeless, she could not see how she could get better at that time and thus the announcement of a longer treatment period did not mean much to her. The only difference, from Zoie's point of view, seemed to be that it was a different label and a more stigmatised one. Zoie watched the film 'Girl, Interrupted' in which the protagonist received the same diagnosis, and got the impression that this new label was highly stigmatizing. She recalled that 'it is probably the second most stigmatised diagnosis after schizophrenia. It is usually associated with perceived "difficult behaviours"'.

This raised the question of whether such a change of diagnosis was helpful for her recovery. Zoie asked the doctor why the diagnosis had changed and was told that the decisive factor was her 'emotional outburst' during her hospital stay. Zoie recalled the incident:

> The visitor's room was very tiny. You know places in Hong Kong are small. During the assigned visiting time, family members would wait in the room to meet the service users. We didn't have privacy. When my husband visited me, sometimes I would lay myself in his embrace or sleep on his shoulder if I was tired. I was not sure if some other visitors officially complained or whether the nurse noticed other people's facial expressions. One day she sternly told me that I could not lay my head on my husband's shoulder. She told me to "behave properly" repeatedly. Feeling very annoyed and thinking that I had done nothing wrong or inappropriately, I yelled back at her. This was the only time I shouted in the hospital, and I thought my reaction was reasonable.

The expression of intimacy towards her husband in the visitor's room was scrutinised with a pathological lens. Zoie's reaction was judged to be 'abnormal' and a 'symptom'. She said, 'No one talked about the incident after that visit. Therefore I am surprised that this incident was written in my report and was considered an evidence of "emotional outburst"'.

Zoie's story is an illustration of the value-laden process of diagnosis and how dependent it is on the contextual power structure. Hospitalisation is considered by clinicians as an opportunity to closely observe service users. Such observation takes place in a highly institutionalised environment, not the context in which service users usually live. This means that service users' behavior is heavily scrutinised in a clinical environment through a lens of 'pathologisation' and what is considered 'appropriate' behaviour is highly value-laden and subjective. However, as Zoie discovered, in a clinical environment, value judgements about what counts as appropriate intimate conduct, can be masked by an 'objective' clinical appearance in a hierarchy of power. Interestingly, Zoie's new diagnosis was changed after two weeks. The psychologist who had known her for many years came back from leave and thought that Zoie was not a case of BPD. The doctor agreed with the psychologist's judgement as she had known Zoie for a long time. Zoie reflected, 'If it was not for her, this highly stigmatised label would have followed me from then on. It was like the psychologist has rescued me from this label'.

The feeling of being 'rescued' revealed Zoie's powerlessness. This powerlessness was a theme that Zoie needed to 'recover from'. The above experience gave Zoie a taste of the way one's behavior could be interpreted and defined as 'abnormal' and one had no say in explaining or defending the behavior. Zoie was articulate and familiar with psychiatric language, yet she could not assert her agency in the context of the acute power disparity in hospital between service users and psychiatrists. This experience had a negative impact on her subsequent help-seeking behavior in the UK. She became acutely aware of how easily what she said and did could be twisted under the psychiatric lens and that it was difficult for service users to assert themselves, especially when they were already in distress. When Zoie had a relapse in the UK, she would ask friends who had knowledge of the local NHS to accompany or help her access the services. She felt that she needed to take great care to make sure what she said was not misinterpreted when seeing members of the medical professional. This was experienced as an extra burden for Zoie and sometimes deterred her from seeking help.

Interventions: what works and what doesn't

Medication is another technology of medicalisation. Medicine was usually the first and often the only treatment option offered to the participants when they first entered the psychiatric services. However, participants said that would have liked to have more options presented and available. Looking back, Ken wished there had been more choices of treatments in Hong Kong. He would have liked to have been offered counselling as he found that it was good to have someone to talk to about his distress. In the UK, where service user movements had been advocating the importance of 'choices', doctors are not usually proactive in giving advice on how service users can help themselves other than prescribing medication. When Carol was asked if doctors suggested any ways to cope when she felt 'out of control', she said they had not. Her doctor only arranged interpretation for her when he needed to prescribe medication. It seems that she was disadvantaged because of the language barriers she faced.

Alongside having no choice of treatment was the possibility that exercising control over one's decision to take medication could be removed. In the experience of some participants starting a course of psychiatric medication did not necessarily come with receiving a diagnosis. Before Marcus experienced a breakdown and his paranoid thoughts resulted in him being sent to the Accident and Emergency Unit of a General Hospital, he suffered from severe headaches. He went to his GP and had a brain scan, but the doctors could not work out the reasons for his headaches. However, the GP prescribed him medication that he found out later was psychiatric medication,

> The doctor didn't tell me what drug it was. He only gave me the medicines in 1 mg doses. I was puzzled. How can 1 mg possibly help me anyway? I only found out that it's a psychiatric drug after I was admitted to the psychiatric hospital.

For Marcus, knowing that it was a psychiatric medication was significant and he was angry for not being told about it. His calling it 'that kind of medication' and implied that it took him a while to digest, accept and decide to take a stigmatised medication. However, the process of digestion and acceptance (or rejection) was not facilitated as the doctor did not explain what was being prescribed and why.

Experience of medications

Does medication help in redeveloping one's mental health capability? Rachel and Lai-Ming recounted how the medications they were prescribed were helpful for them to maintain daily functioning. Rachel, diagnosed with schizophrenia, saw medication as an important element in maintaining her daily life on her recovery journey. Lai-Ming was on heavy medication and injections for nearly 40 years. Although he had side effects such as muscle spasm and sleepiness, he tolerated them as he thought 'the medication keeps me going. Mostly I am well'. Nin-Jin described finding the right medication as being one of the important turning points of her recovery after several rounds of psychotic episodes.

Other participants expressed reservations about their medication. Ken was prescribed an antidepressant and an antipsychotic for his delusions and paranoia, together with a neurological medication to stop his leg shaking. He said he now understood why people did not like taking psychiatric medication.

> The medication makes you feel bad. Taking it makes you feel like . . . becoming another person. You feel like time flies very slowly. I took a bus from one terminus to and fro the other terminus just to kill the time, to make time pass easier . . . I cannot concentrate. I felt like I was "clouded", deprived of all kind of emotions. Like the emotions were being suppressed.

Feng was told that the anti-psychotic drug he was taking did not have side effects. He did not believe it, 'It's not possible that it has no side effects. Taking this medication made me dependent on it. If you stop it, you can't control your mind. It becomes dependency. You can't stop the medication. You have to take it'.

Some side effects seem to be capability diminishing. They could affect participants immediately and/or have an impact on their outlook on life and their life plans. Carol said her doctor warned her that the tranquillisers she was on would result in her having dementia around the age of 40. Zoie was not prepared to carry on taking the medication that she had started taking in her twenties. She experienced withdrawal symptoms when trying to come off it under the doctor's guidance. She had read that the medication she was on would be harmful to a foetus if she became pregnant. Now in her thirties, she had to factor in the risk of withdrawal, changing medication and relapse when considering whether to have a baby.

It could take a long time for service users and their doctors to find the right dosage and mix of medicines. Some participants found that this period could be very confusing. For example, the side effects of psychiatric medication could be similar to the symptoms that it was supposed to control. Carol was diagnosed with 'post-natal depression'. When she started her medication, she was prescribed an antidepressant and a antipsychotic drug and said the medications had given her very bad side effects, 'That one really drives me crazy. A sane person will become insane! It was too strong. I did not know which one caused me more suffering, this medicine or the illness'.

Similarly, a quick increase of her antidepressants pushed Zoie over the edge. The agitation that resulted made her suicidal urges unbearable. For Zoie, this experience was traumatic. She admitted herself to hospital and the hospitalisation marked a turning point in her life. The memory of her extreme distress and vulnerability became something that Zoie had to recover from on her recovery journey.

Participants could not get a clear answer from their doctors about their experiences of symptoms and side effects. Feng's active quest to understand his distress and the medication he was prescribed was dismissed. Feng made an appointment with his GP to talk about his obsessive worry over daily matters and whether it was a side effect of his prescribed anti-psychotic. However, the GP did not give him an answer nor did he advise Feng about ways to cope with his obsessive worry. Instead he just told Feng to keep taking the medication. The side effects participants complained about were, they claimed, not always taken seriously. They said they did not get satisfactory answers from clinicians. Often, they thought their concerns about side effects were viewed by doctors as signs of non-compliance.

Whether to stay on medications or not: agency and coercion

For these participants, the decisions they made about whether to stay on medication or not was a matter of weighing the pros and cons. They had to decide whether the medications helped and whether the side effects were worth tolerating. They would consider significant others, the association between medication and patienthood, as well as the causes of their distress. Through this 'weighing-up exercise' participants demonstrated how they wanted to assert agency in their use of medication in their recovery.

This process is not often acknowledged or facilitated by the professionals. In situations where medications were forced upon participants they felt a continuing sense of victimhood and grievance. Raymond could not work out if his prescribed medication was helping him or not. During regular medical checks for his disabling heart condition, Raymond told his GP that he felt hopeless as nothing was progressing in his life and he had written a suicide note. He was prescribed antidepressants. He did not ask for medication but his GP thought he needed it. He stopped taking it as he felt it was not helping him. Nearly all the participants who were on long-term medication organised a cessation on a trial and error basis, with or without letting the doctors know. For doctors, such behaviour was often considered to be going against medical advice. Some participants, like Feng, found their queries about medication were dismissed and so decided to take matters into their own hands and experiment with trying to see how they could cope without medication. For some, this experience resulted in an acceptance of medication. For example, Feng and Ken both tried stopping their medication to test out if they would be all right without it. They found that their old symptoms returned. This convinced Feng that he needed medication. Ken thought that he 'had to' accept taking the medication, although it did not 'cure' him or his paranoia. He described himself as living 'under its shadow', and reacted to people who looked suspicious to him.

Some participants took their medications for the sake of significant others. Having had several breakdowns, Wu-Wei decided to keep taking her medication out of consideration to her family.

> If I don't take the medication, my family that I treasure very much would be destroyed. I am not just me. I am also a mother. Most important is that I am a mother. Also my husband loves me very much. And I love this family. If anything happened to me, who could take care of the children if my husband were at work? My in-laws would step in to help, but I did not want to be looked down on by them. So I have to be strong.

She had a strong incentive to keep taking her medication, which was fuelled by her 'mission' to be a good mother and stay strong in front of her in-laws. Despite this strong motivation, she was still ambivalent about the idea of taking medications long term and tried to reduce her dosage secretly.

Wu-Wei: I don't want to take so many pills for the rest of my life.
Author: Do you accept that you have to be on medication forever?
Wu-Wei: Maybe I don't accept this. Taking medication keeps reminding me I am a mental patient.

Medication brought the unwanted side-product of patienthood that Wu-Wei found difficult to shake off. Patienthood, associated with long-term medication, became a burden that Wu-Wei needed to recover from. While taking medications enabled her to fulfill her mothering role, which helped improve her self-esteem, patienthood added a dimension of struggle against passive victimhood.

Compared to other participants, Tang-Yung was still uncertain about whether her medication helped her. Her medication was changed to injections because her doctor thought she might throw her medication away. The medication were said to curb her spending urge to buy clothes, which resulted in her debts. However, she did not think she was ill, 'I don't want to take medication, because I think my problem is a financial problem. Not this mental illness problem. Because there are things I couldn't solve'.

She felt that her life had crumbled after the burglary of her possessions at the time she was building a life away from her husband. Because of the setback, she started to become obsessive about buying clothes. Having been on the injection for a long time, she could not tell if the medication helped her or made her feel worse as she found it difficult to control her emotions. She gained weight as a result of the medication and this upset her further as she could not wear the pretty clothes she liked. She expressed contempt for the way her medication was forced upon her and this added to her grievances.

Enabling factors for managing medication: within and outside medical encounters

What are the enabling factors that empower service users to make decisions about taking medication in ways that contribute to the redevelopment of their mental well-being? As shown in Feng's narrative, doctors who take a patronising attitude to service users' concern about the side effects of their medication do not help tackle doubts about medication. A lack of explanation from a doctor can also reflect social class, ethnic differences and language barriers. A comparison between Zoie and Nin-Jin's experiences illustrated further the importance of doctors exploring medications together with service users – what Deegan and Drake (2006) call a 'shared decision-making' model in medical management against medical paternalism.

When Zoie sought help from her GP for a relapse in the UK, she was very reluctant to follow the doctor's advice to increase the dosage of her medication. This was because of the bad experience she had when changing dosage in her previous breakdown. She also worried about the difficulties she would have reducing the dosage in the future. Later she was referred to a psychiatrist who did not rush to increase her dosage. He listened to her concerns and agreed to take time and explore if she really needed to increase the dosage as suggested by the GP. Zoie thought that taking her concerns and her past experience on board as well as taking the necessary time to investigate the medicines together was helpful in maintaining her agency in managing medication and respecting the experiences she had accumulated through her years of taking medication.

In contrast, Nin-Jin's felt that her past experience of using medication was ignored by her doctor. She had expressed strong reservations about changing her medication when her new psychiatrist wanted her to stop taking one of her pills. She was given no reasons for this change to her prescription and she was not asked for her opinion about the proposed reduction.

> I said I couldn't reduce it. He did not believe in me. I followed his instruction. And then I really felt very ill! . . . I am not sure if it's because he doesn't understand me or what. It was a huge psychological threat, reducing the medicine like that. I had been doing fine before that.

She was clearly upset and reported feeling ill after complying with the doctor's advice. Reducing medicine felt, in her words, to be a 'psychological threat' to her because she was the one who had to live with the consequences of 'having the boat rocked' – a boat in which she for many years had tried to stay afloat.

This comparison of experiences shows not only the importance of empowering service users in a context of medical dominance. It is crucial to recognise the value of service users' knowledge of their own health and experience of the effect of medication on them. Both Zoie and Nin-Jin had been on medication for a long time and had accumulated valuable experience about their conditions. Language barriers and social class seem to be significant in explaining the differing experiences of Zoie, Feng and Nin-Jin. As a university graduate who spoke fluent English and was knowledgeable about psychiatric terminology Zoie did not rely on interpreters like Feng and Nin-Jin. This suggests that social class differences influence the extent that doctors are willing to offer explanations (Pendleton and Bochner, 1980).

The social class distance between clinicians and service users can adversely impact on the building of rapport if clinicians are not reflexive about their class positions. To enable service users to actively manage their medication, a shared decision-making approach to counter medical dominance would also be needed to tackle power disparities arising from social class differences and language barriers. Here, 'value-based practice', in which the professionals take account of the difference of values between them and service users, might be useful in facilitating recovery without compromising service users' agency. A reduction in disagreement resulting from power disparity could be achieved if the preferences and concerns the service user brings to medical encounters are integrated into decision-making about their recovery plan (Fulford and Wallcraft, 2009).

Aside from the realm of medical encounters, participants' narratives revealed that significant others as well as Chinese community centres sometimes had a role in participants' use of medication in their recovery journeys. The role of family members can be both positive and negative in assisting service users to incorporate medication in their recovery journeys.

Rachel felt that it was helpful for her mother to remind her to take her medications if she forgot to do so. However, in some cases, family members' opinion on the medications could be a source of stress for participants. Jerry's parents held different opinions to him about his medication plan and complained to the doctor if the dosage was not reduced over time. Jerry as an adult did not have a problem with his prescribed medication. Yet, he was stressed because of his parents' opinions. Parents could expand an individual's capability, as Rachel discovered, but Jerry's parents denied him agency.

Chinese-speaking workers with knowledge about psychiatric medication in Chinese community centres could assist service users' understanding of their prescriptions. Lai-Ming had found help from such a worker useful as he could talk to the worker whenever he had a query about his medication problems. Such workers provided something that doctors might not provide. Although Lai-Ming could speak fluent English, talking to a worker with the same first language gave him a feeling of 'brotherhood'. It was different from seeing a doctor when one was ill. This worker was like a friend from whom Lai-Ming could seek advice for anything that troubled him.

Experiences of talking therapy

Alongside medication, talking therapy was mentioned as an intervention that participants had used. Half of the participants had used psychological services from the statutory or voluntary sector. Some participants did not like talking therapy. Rachel did not consider it as an option because she did not like to discuss her illness. Two participants had tried counselling but did not think the experience helped because they thought the counsellor or therapist did not understand them. Raymond was referred to the counselling at his GP practice after revealing that he felt hopeless living with his disabling heart problem. He had two sessions with the counsellor and then stopped. He thought the experience was 'pointless', as he did not think the counsellor understood him. Jerry thought that the psychological therapy he had had could not help him with the spiritual problems that preoccupied him. He preferred going to his church for pastoral care and spiritual discussion. It is worth noting that Rachel, Raymond and Jerry were born or grew up in the UK, spoke perfect English and at the same time had been brought up in a Chinese environment created by their first-generation migrant parents. This points to the need for further research on whether 'not being understood' and 'not wanting to talk about illness' are linked to a lack of understanding of the experiences of British born Chinese people (Parker and Song, 2007).

Five participants had used Chinese-speaking counselling services arranged by Chinese community centres in the UK. Some of these participants, especially those who had been overseas brides and could not speak fluent English, considered that talking therapy was very important in their recovery. Having someone to talk to about their distress and troubles was a major reason for them using these services. Abao, Bai-Xin and Carol recommended talking therapy highly and thought that it should be made widely available to Chinese people.

Talking therapy was found to be capability enhancing for these participants because they had no one else to talk to about their discontent with life in the UK. This partly reflects the barriers they experienced because of their limited

English speaking skills and their lack of local Chinese friends. They would nod and chat with other Chinese people, for example in Chinatown, but said they were more like acquaintances than understanding friends who they could talk to. Fear of gossip was another reason that deterred them from casually revealing themselves to other Chinese people. They did not feel able to talk to their families and friends in their home country, as they did not want them to worry. They thought that their families and friends at home might not be able to understand their problems living in the UK.

Bai-Xin recalled the cathartic effect for her of counselling. Before going to counselling, she felt unable to cry despite her deep distress, 'I didn't look like a human being. I didn't know who I am'. She felt much better after crying. For Abao, counselling provided a space for her to vent her frustration and stress as a full-time carer for a husband with learning difficulties and her three children. The caring responsibilities took a toll on her for many years and it affected her relationship with her children. Having someone to reveal this stress to, in confidence, transformed her. It increased her capability to deal with her own frustration and face the guilt she felt, as well as her capability to parent and relate to her daughter. This benefitted both her and her family. She felt tremendous relief and learnt communication skills from the counsellor. She was able to talk to her daughters calmly as a result. She also learnt how to manage her stress when she felt her temper was going to get the better of her. As discussed in Chapter 3, she had not considered that she should take proper care of herself in the past. Now she would take a short walk from home when her stress mounted, realising that it was important that she took care of herself so that she was in a good state to look after her household.

Talking therapy can facilitate the development of skills to cope with distress. It can help service users develop their capabilities to deal with distress and function in their daily lives. It gives power to service users to deal with the difficult emotions they experience. For some participants this sense of agency would not have been gained by just taking medication. Carol and Wu-Wei had been hospitalised and were on long-term medication. They found the self-understanding they learnt through counselling very useful in enabling them to feel in control of their ill health. Carol used the Chinese-speaking telecounselling services. The telecounselling services suited Carol's need for a flexible schedule in case she was unable to leave the house for her appointment because of her panic attacks. She did not think that not seeing the counsellor face to face was a hindrance as she found she had developed a good therapeutic relationship with the counsellor over the phone.

While counselling could be cathartic, the process could be challenging. Carol's counsellor told her at the first session that the process could be hard so Carol felt prepared. She was able to work through repressed issues since childhood with the counsellor and started to recognise what triggered her panic attacks. Over time her ability to understand her own emotions increased. For Wu-Wei, the counselling she had in the UK was the first time she had the opportunity to talk to someone about her sexual abuse as a child in mainland China. The counselling increased her awareness of the signs of feeling emotionally unwell and what she could do to calm herself. She learnt skills, such as meditation, to take care of herself. Increased self-esteem was another important outcome shared by Abao, Bai-Xin and Carol after the talking therapy. Carol felt more confident in general.

> The counsellor helped me to be able to have conversations with other people and to have contact with society again. Because of this illness, you have low-esteem. You also lack confidence. Of course it's not a stable progress, but at least I feel that I am becoming more like a human being again.

For Abao and Bai-Xin, counselling enabled them to become more involved in the activities of the Chinese community centre. Their increased self-esteem improved their capability to connect with the community (Ware *et al.*, 2007).

Enabling factors for using talking therapy

Zoie and Carol had tried several therapists in Hong Kong and the UK. They both considered it was not easy to find the 'right' one and could tell when they could 'connect with' a therapist, e.g. whether they were able to cry in the presence of the therapist. Carol was conscious of retaining control when she started a new therapy.

> I tell you, for illness like this, not all counsellors suit you. Because for sensitive people like us, you hear a single word or phrase . . . A single word can make you relapse. It's a protection to myself. It took a lot of time for me to get used to a new therapist. It took a lot of energy to tell the new person your history. It did not guarantee that we could get along.

Carol and Zoie had clear ideas about what they thought a good counsellor or therapist was like.

Carol: My counsellor is really professional. She is very skillful in talking to the clients. She wouldn't agitate you, nor just sit there to listen to you. She makes you feel comfortable and not embarrassed, and leads you to say what you want to say.

Zoie: You can feel that the therapist is genuinely interested in you. She would not dismiss your disagreement with what she said is your 'defence mechanism'.

While many participants considered talking therapy important for their recovery journeys, its cost and availability were factors that could limit access. Funding available for talking therapy and for training Chinese-speaking counsellors is vital to making therapy accessible. Zoie said that she could not have afforded private therapy if her psychiatrist had not referred her for NHS therapy. Chinese community centres were the main sources of help for participants needing a Chinese-speaking counsellor. However, Chinese counselling services are not always available. If the local NHS had good links with Chinese community centres service users would be referred to them. Wu-Wei was referred to a Chinese counselling service when she was discharged from hospital. Otherwise she might not have known about talking therapy and how to access it. In areas where Chinese community centres were small, counselling services were less embedded. Funding was sporadic, resulting in interruptions to the services and a loss of counsellors when funding finished.

Hospitalisation

Voluntary and compulsory admission

The process of hospital admission and being an inpatient emerged as the central experiences of psychiatric power for participants. Whether the experience of hospitalisation was a capability enhancing experience was closely related to a number of factors: the pathway to hospitalisation; whether participants could speak the national language; engagement with fellow service users and whether treatments were forced upon participants against their will during the stay. Of the participants, 12 out of 22 had experiences of hospitalisation. Some had been admitted more than once. Ten had been admitted to UK psychiatric hospitals; three of their admissions had been involuntarily. All three participants admitted in mainland China were sent there by their families on an involuntary basis. Of the five participants admitted in Hong Kong, one was admitted involuntarily.

Some participants could not recall the process of admission because of the distress they were experiencing. Some had made a choice to go to hospital. Wu-Wei recalled that having been forced to go, in her words, to 'dodgy' hospitals in mainland China, she was willing to go to a UK hospital as she considered it a 'proper hospital'. Nin-Jia agreed to go to hospital because she was feeling very unwell, and having tried drinking 'talisman' she felt she needed to believe in something 'real'. But still she considered going to the hospital was an option where there were no others available. Not all the decisions about voluntary admission were made wholeheartedly. It is well documented that some service users go into hospital voluntarily, not because they want to but because they are threatened with being sectioned if they do not go (Hoge *et al.*, 1997; Pescosolido *et al.*, 1998).

Jerry agreed to voluntary admission in the UK to avoid being sectioned. He thought that social workers could be 'troublesome' if you did not agree to what they suggested. He chose to be admitted voluntarily to prevent having to deal with mental health laws, which he was not familiar with. This decision was about avoiding trouble rather than making an agreement about what would help him. It encapsulated the acute power inequality that service users experience and the lack of capability to exercise their rights. Such forced 'voluntary' admissions are not about exercising agency – they reflect a diminishment of capability.

The process of compulsory admission is not capability enhancing because it denies agency. The denial of agency during a compulsory admission could become an experience some participants had to recover from later on in their recovery journeys. There was one exception, a participant for whom compulsory admission provided a marked improvement in his mental state and support that he could not have accessed otherwise. He considered that compulsory admission had stopped his mental health capability from further diminishment and deterioration. After Feng left his job in the restaurant, his mental health deteriorated severely. He attempted suicide at home, refused to see people and suffered psychotic experiences. The worker who introduced me to Feng said she was present when he was sectioned and his admission was dramatic and chaotic. In retrospect, Feng said he really was ill at that time. This acceptance of his compulsory admission might have been the result of his marked improvement during his hospital stay. He rapidly received care as a result of hospitalisation. The increase of the quality and intensity of the interventions available to him after hospitalisation reflected his extremely vulnerable position as an undocumented migrant. As an undocumented immigrant he did not have access to NHS services. After hospitalisation, he could access statutory mental health services and support. At the same time, he started to apply for asylum seeker status and was thus able to receive one year of continual care after discharge.

However, a number of participants expressed strong grievances about compulsory admission. Tang-yung said she felt tricked into a psychiatric hospital by her family in mainland China. Since then she had lost trust in her family. Wu-Wei was taken to hospital in mainland China about 10 years ago when she was in in her early twenties. She strongly disapproved of the hospital. Because she had been compulsorily admitted, she could not reject the treatment forced on her. She described the electroconvulsive therapy that she had to administer herself: 'Every day I had to queue up for electrocution. There was a machine and I had to take an electrical wire to electrocute myself. It is still a nightmare to me. I felt very scared'.

Carol described the detrimental effect that compulsory hospitalisation in the UK had had on her. She felt that the process of the involuntary admission was traumatic. At first she actively sought help for her overwhelming mental distress, but the result was far from empowering. This bad experience deterred her from seeking help and having trust in the mental health services. Carol developed acute post-natal depression soon after giving birth to her son in Hong Kong. The depression got worse when she returned to the UK to rejoin her husband. She was very exhausted and was scared by her intrusive thoughts of harming her baby. She struggled not to act on these thoughts.

> I put him on the sofa and then locked myself in the kitchen. I threw the keys into the garden so that I won't be able to pick them up. I called my husband. I said something really happened to me and he really needed to come home right away.

Carol was in great distress and worried that she would hurt her son. At the same time, she took measures to keep herself from acting out her ideations and actively asked for help. Her husband took her to see the GP who told her to calm down and go home to wait for the emergency team. A nurse and a doctor came and replaced the medications she was prescribed in Hong Kong. She was told to try the different medication but its functions and possible side effects were not discussed with her. Carol began to feel worse and did not know whether this was the side effects of the drugs or a deterioration in her health. Apart from medication, the emergency team did not offer her advice about coping with her distressing thoughts or provide any practical help about taking care of the baby. Instead, they forced her to go to the hospital. She recalled that the doctor and the social worker had different opinions about whether she could cope at home. The doctor told her that 99.9 per cent of the mothers with post-natal depression would not hurt their baby. He thought Carol could handle it. But the social worker did not agree. Carol was hospitalised involuntarily in a mother and baby unit for 2 months, which seem to add to her distress.

> They used power to force me to go to the hospital. I cried every day in the hospital, because I had a deep grievance. Why didn't you give me the rights as a patient not to go to the hospital? Why did you force me? Every time I had a meeting with the social worker, the doctor and the interpreter in the hospital, I was very agitated. No matter how I saw it, I was much less crazy than the other five people in the ward. Because every day I had to face those people, who cut themselves and lost lots of blood or kept escaping from the ward, I will really became crazy, wouldn't you?

Carol got very angry as she recounted this episode. Instead of trying to figure out an arrangement to help the whole family, she felt that the social worker was more concerned with the safety of the baby than helping her. Her husband was allowed to be present during her assessment but not allowed to interpret for her. While it could be argued that not using a family member as an informal interpreter was to protect the confidentiality and privacy of the service user, especially in situation where family member is linked to the crisis of the user (Costa, 2013), the interpreter arranged by the doctor was not competent in Carol's view. Carol thought the interpreter's poor performance contributed to the decision to force her to go to hospital, 'She said I wanted to kill him! [Her baby son] But ideations and actions are two different matters! She translated it wrong but I could do nothing about this'.

Carol actively asked for help. It was her first contact with the UK mental health services, but her agency was invalidated. She felt that she was not trusted. I asked if there were anything that the hospital did right for her. Carol thought that one thing the hospital did right was that they forced her to bond with the baby, to face the reality that he was born. I asked if there were any midwives or nurses who helped her with the bonding at home, she said no. This experience of involuntary admission had an adverse impact of Carol's help-seeking later on.

Carol clearly articulated her experiences of power disparity and helplessness when using mental health services. This negative experience diminished her confidence in using these services actively and cooperatively. What she needed to recover from, after her involuntary admission, was her loss of trust in the services. Yet, it seems that her grievances were never acknowledged and reconciliation was not facilitated.

Her post-natal depression developed into a long-term mental health problem that she had to cope with every day. She became a long-term service user, but contact with the services was a burden to her. The compulsory hospitalisation had made her become resentful and fearful of the mental health services and resulted in her losing faith in them. Her bad experience made her weary with psychiatric services during her second pregnancy, in which she had a long relapse and very distressing symptoms. This time she experienced suicidal thoughts. Although she was certain that she would not act on them, these suicidal urges were painful and impairing. The mental health trust sent her letters about the prenatal services. Instead of seeing these appointments as a support to help her through the pregnancy, she thought that they were just 'being ready to "catch" her'. 'They just wanted to control me. This only gave me more pressure. I can't see how they can help me. I can't see how keeping me in the hospital or visiting me can help me.'

She had the same feeling towards asking for help from social services. She did not want a social worker and did not like the idea of having a key worker or support worker to help her with household chores or taking care of her son. Although in theory a social worker and key worker could have flexibly accommodated her needs, over the years of using the services, she was not shown how alternative arrangements could possibly help. Carol changed from being a person who actively sought help from services into a 'service avoider'.

Hospital life

Sorting out a medication regime under close observation is one of the reasons participants were admitted to inpatient units. Their narratives about whether hospitalisation was considered helpful for recovery highlighted how the relationships they built with other service users were treasured. Rachel was transferred to an inpatient unit from the outpatient clinic of the hospital in the UK. She found the hospital stay helpful because it helped with her medication. Language capability, i.e. being able to speak English, and her prior contact with community-based mental health services contributed to her good experience in the hospital. It enhanced the redevelopment of her mental health well-being.

Getting along with other patients was another reason some participants found hospitalisation a positive experience. The relationships, even friendships, which developed with other service users, gave some participants a sense of community that was constructive for recovering their mental well-being. The exchange of skills and mutual learning that could happen in such community could be capability developing. When Lai-Ming stayed in an open ward in Hong Kong, he walked around freely, and enjoyed exercise such as playing badminton with fellow service users. Similarly, as a teenager in mainland China, Hins enjoyed chatting with fellow service users in the hospital.

We shared the same misery. Actually it was good. They knew a lot of things and taught me a lot of things. I have a vivid memory of one woman . . . After the nurse turned off the light, we would lie beside each other and chat.

Yet, some participants did not find the hospital a place of safety or sanctuary. For Jerry and Marcus, this was not due to language problems as they could speak English very well. The institutionalisation process uprooted them from their usual living environments and feelings of estrangement added to their distress. They did not find hospitalisation therapeutic. Jerry recalled his first stay in a psychiatric hospital in the UK as a young adult. Although he was born in the UK, the experience was akin to a 'cultural shock'.

It was frightening. I've never seen such a poverty of . . . It was very basic. Everything was basic. It frightened me. Before the stay, my mom and dad had been looking after me. Now I was in hospital. They couldn't help me. And I had all these unnatural thoughts . . . It was frightening.

Marcus said being in the hospital was 'really not fun at all'.

Marcus: You don't really notice when you first got in. But after a few days it started to sink in. For example, the food is different from what you eat outside. The ward is a square box . . . I was pacing around in the box. Pacing around. I felt suicidal.
Author: Because of the setting of the ward?
Marcus: I don't know. I didn't know what contributed to the painful feeling. Anyway I felt suicidal inside but other people can't see that. Then I was allowed home.

Some participants who faced a language barrier used isolation to counter hospitalisation. Preoccupied with unwanted thoughts, Feng hid himself in his own room. Basic English language skills and simple words alongside gestures were enough when a stay was relatively 'uneventful'. Nin-Jin felt that the hospital provided a sense of safety and the medical staff were experienced and understood her problems. She even made a few friends there. In cases where service users were more outspoken and outgoing, language barriers could cause problems.

Oa-Yang's experiences illustrated how her inability to explain herself in English resulted in her resorting to unconventional ways of protecting herself and communicating. Such unconventional ways crossed the line of normality/abnormality laid down by the hospital. She didn't say whether her various hospital stays were voluntary or not. She recounted times when she felt desperate and laid a knife on her skin, and times when her husband wanted her to go to the hospital as she was 'out of control'. She said she got along well with most of the other service users in the hospital, teaching them Chinese. Oa-Yang was used to resolving conflicts and 'restoring justice' by beating people up. She had used self-defence with her fists since childhood. She learnt that to be discharged she had to curb her outgoing character and stop being violent.

> They didn't let me go even when I was recovered. I wanted to file a lawsuit against them. The doctor said I didn't need to. He would let me go in two-week's time. It turned out that they kept me for 6 months. I figured out a plan. I went upstairs to the elderly ward, I helped clean them up. Wiped their faces. Combed their hair. Took them to the toilets. If they saw how good I was and thought that I had recovered, that I wasn't mad, I thought they would let me out. But they didn't. So I sat there. Sitting there all the time, dozing.

Through these experiences Oa-Yang learnt about the behaviours that were considered 'normal' by professionals.

Author: What was the situation when they let you out of hospital?
Oa-Yang: When I became normal again.
Author: How do you become normal?
Oa-Yang: Not singing or playing kungfu. Not beating people up. Not raising my fists and feet. Then they let me go.'

However, she said she still beat people up because the nurses did not intervene when she was beaten by other service users and she had to defend herself. The following quote shows that her 'grandiose' ideas and 'abnormal' thinking were symbolic. She did not know how to explain the symbolism in English and sometimes did not bother to be understood.

Oa-Yang: Some people are scared of me. That's the problem.
Author: Why would they be scared of you?
Oa-Yang: Because I am Queen of the gang [a title she said she got when being in the gangster circles when young].
Author: But new people you meet don't know your title.
Oa-Yang: They think that I am mad. That's the problem.
Author: Do you explain to them?
Oa-Yang: I don't know how to explain. So I can only say I am a fish.
Author: But this will further encourage people to believe that you are mad.
Oa-Yang: That's the problem. But I really am a fish. I told people in the hospital that I am a fish. Because fish is the most clever, but also the most forgetful. That's why I am a 'forgetful fish'. Haha. [*Shi Yun Yu* or forgetful fish is a Cantonese expression that means one is a forgetful and mindless soul.]
Author: If you don't explain to people, people don't understand what you mean by 'forgetful fish'.
Oa-Yang: So now I am explaining to you.
Author: If you meet new people and tell them you are a fish, they will think you are mad.

Oa-Yang: Yes indeed. Because 1,000 years ago I am a fish, now I am a human being. Now I am human being, not a fish. That's why.
Author: Some people may not have the patience to listen to your explanation.
Oa-Yang: Yes, that's why they will die. Their whole family will cease.
Author: Those who don't listen to you will die?
Oa-Yang: Yes. They have illness.
Author: That will scare people away.
Oa-Yang: So don't tell people about this. They will be scared. Don't tell the children. Because I love them very much.

As this exchange illustrated what seemed unintelligible could be understood. Two comments on the intersection of psychiatric pathologisation and ethnicity can be made here. First, as in Zoie's experience of a changed diagnosis because she shouted at a nurse, Oa-Yang's experience showed that an individual's behavior in a hospital institution is scrutinised primarily under the lens of pathologisation and ab/normality. The meanings behind what service users say or do not say is not often taken into account. Second, pathologisation intersected with the disadvantages Oa-Yang faced as a member of a non-English speaking ethnic minority. The cultural insensitivity of professionals is due to language barriers as well as a lack of knowledge about symbolic meanings in different cultures. If a practitioner attempts to work with meanings, a wealth of knowledge about the repertoire of symbolism, myths and colloquialisms in different languages and cultures would be required to achieve a sufficient understanding to work with service users from different cultural backgrounds. Having practitioners who can speak the same language is important as they can talk to service users without the mediation of an interpreter. However, it should not be assumed that multilingual staff are necessarily knowledgeable about cultural repertoires as cultural 'heritage' is fluid. The regional dialects of different Chinese communities, within China or overseas, are constantly invented and reinvented. Similarly, the fluidity of 'cultural meanings' crisscrosses with gender and class. The gender and class background of professionals can affect their sensitivity to the needs and articulations of service users with a different background. This indicates the need for an intersectional approach rather than using culturalist assumption in developing the cultural sensitivity practitioners and institutions need.

   Having shared participants' accounts of their experiences of different elements of medicalisation, i.e. diagnosis, different forms of treatment and hospitalisation and their negative and positive impact on their mental health capabilities, the ways that participants reflected on the process as a whole is now explored. If mental distress and ill health are considered as a kind of crisis resulting in chaos and paralysis in life, the question needs to be asked about the ways that the medicalisation of distress can enable service users to make sense of crises and develop understandings that help them regain a control and orient their lives. Nin-Jin's story is used to illustrate the 'incomplete' project of medicalisation and how it opens up the possibility of agency development using cultural resources in understanding distress and ill health.

The 'incomplete' project of medicalisation and pragmatism in adopting explanatory models

The story of Nin-Jin illustrated the importance of meaning-making in one's recovery journey and how the domination of bio-medical discourse did not facilitate the process of meaning-making. When the worker from a Chinese community centre referred Nin-Jin to me, she told me that she was glad that Nin-Jin had finally accepted that she had a mental illness. However, Nin-Jin's narrative showed that it was an acceptance of the role of medication in maintaining a balanced mental state that enabled her to carry on daily life that she longed for, instead of her acceptance of having a mental illness. In fact, co-existing explanatory models of medicalisation and possession by the devil was shown in her narratives (Kleinman *et al.*, 1978). The co-existing explanatory models were constituted through a pragmatic 'trial and error' process, epitomised in her use of the phrase 'I cannot not believe in' when talking about the two explanatory models.

At first, Nin-Jin could not sleep and had been constantly disturbed by nightmares when she started to feel ill. She was scared of people and her surrounding, describing a feeling of being 'disturbed by dirty things'. 'Dirty things' is a euphemism in Chinese language for ghosts. It should be emphasised here that a 'disturbance by ghosts' is one of (instead of the sole) cultural resources/ideologies that Chinese participants draw upon to explain suffering. Feng and Wu-Wei, for example, were adamant about their disbelief in the existence of ghosts. Nin-Jin thought that not being able to adjust to life in the UK contributed to her ill health. Her family in Hong Kong worshipped Taoist Gods and took her to pray in a Taoist temple where she was given 'talismanic medicine' to drink. It did not make her feel better. Some friends suggested that she should find a medium to exorcise her. She was suspicious of this because some other friends said the medium was a cheat. 'I mean I should believe in real things, instead of those that aren't. Those ghostly things seem fake. I prefer to believe in a doctor.'

It took a long time for Nin-Jin to attain a stable mental state and she did feel ill. She thought there had been two important turning points in her recovery. One important turning point was getting the right medication. She did not believe she had a mental illness and thought the doctors had made a mistake until she felt significantly better after taking the right medication. She felt calmer and more peaceful after taking it. When she tried not to take them, she felt ill right away. Since then she 'accepted' that she 'had a mental illness', because she had tested the effect of not taking the medicine. As she put it, 'I cannot *not* believe it is a mental illness'.

The second turning point for Nin-Jin was finding Christian religion. In the past she believed in and worshipped KwanYin. Although she described the Taoist model of exorcism as 'unreal', she said exorcism by a Christian church helped her instantly feel better. It was a spiritual journey that resembled a sudden calling, one that she described as a 'miracle'.

I don't know why. Something within me urged me to go to Church. I went to one church. I don't know anything about that church at that time, not in Hong Kong or in the UK. Somehow I found it. It was like a sixth sense. I was surprised too. They found a Chinese-speaking vicar to help me. They helped me exorcise the devil. Help me remove it. The devil disturbed me, but there is also a positive spirit that helped me. I felt that these two both existed inside me.

Her account of 'being possessed' seems to be contradictory. Nin-Jin thought she should not believe in the Taoist model of possession by 'dirty things', but she believed in the Christian model of exorcism. She said that 'ghostly things seem fake' and thought she should believe in the doctor. However, she believed that she was indeed possessed. 'I *believe* in both. I *believe* I have devil in me. I also *believe* that I am ill. Anyway I know that I *felt* ill. The medication does help me. So I *know* that I have an illness' (emphasis by author). These seeming contradictions made sense in the context of the trial and error of a recovery journey as experienced by service users.

Author: How did you explain the devil possession?
Nin-Jin: Christianity believes in the devil as well. It's not only Taoist temples that believe in it. Christianity believes in it too and they use their methods to exorcise it. I am surprised that it was quite good. Eating the talismanic medicine is not as powerful as the Christian method.

It was not abstract belief systems that constituted her explanatory models. Instead, her understanding of her ill health was constituted pragmatically, i.e. what worked and what did not work for her. The explanatory models an individual adopts are constituted, verified and reformulated accordingly throughout the recovery process. Service users will pick up the cultural resources available to them in the process of sense-making.

Although Nin-Jin was able to pinpoint two turning points in her recovery journey, during the interview she kept asking me what I thought the reasons were for her mental ill health. She gave me several possible reasons for her distress, e.g. her dislike of living in the UK after 30 years, post-natal problems, the stress of raising children on her own, but these did not seem to be a satisfactory explanation to her. She was familiar with the explanation offered by the bio-medical model, 'it was a lack of chemical in the brain and therefore one has to take medicine to supplement it'. Yet 'why has this happened to me' was a question that she kept bringing up in the interview. Nin-Jin's comment on her family's reaction to her ill health provided some insight into this, 'They don't understand me. I guess they think everybody is fine apart from me'.

The 'sick role' status sanctioned by medicalisation may offer a temporary relief space for some service users and provide legitimacy for getting help from health and social services and medication. However, it creates a demarcation of 'normal' and 'abnormal' that encourages self-stigmatisation, which is capability diminishing, and doesn't help develop understanding from others. Positive usage of non-biomedical discourses then seems to facilitate recovery in the sense of narrating a positive sense of self that is crucial in agency development.

Conclusions

This chapter has demonstrated that the transnational context is important in the pathway to care. Some participants who were migrants used health care in their home countries and were enabled to recover a mental state that supported their daily functioning. However, such use of transnational health care could be disempowering when coercion was involved. Seeking help from health care services on a recovery journey was revealed as a trial and error process, with turning points when individuals found out what worked for them and what did not. Facilitating and supporting service users to explore what works is therefore important if they are to take control of their recovery journeys.

In this regard, the application of Capability Approaches has two important dimensions. First, the negative experiences of this process of seeking medical help should not be understood as a 'trade off' or 'necessary evil'. The multi-dimensional development of capabilities and agency of service users should be supported. Second, the centrality of agency in the Capabilities Approach enables an understanding of agency in the recovery process.

The importance of exercising agency goes beyond a vague ideal. It is central to recovery as a capability-enhancing process:

> The capabilities approach explicitly allows for – in fact, it affirmatively *builds in* – a tension between well-being (being well provided for) and agency (pursuing one's own life projects and cultivating self-respect (original emphasis) . . . To put it bluntly: *agency* is not only the wounded faculty ostensibly being treated; it also conditions – that is, it enables, constrains and shapes – how effective care and basic securities are provided at all.
>
> (Hopper 2009: 13)

Agency is not a value judgement. As Hopper rightly puts it, foregrounding service user agency is a condition in which care should be provided and received. Close scrutiny is necessary when decisions are made about whether a person 'lacks' capacity and is 'in need of protection' against their expressed intentions. At such times question have to be asked about the alternatives available in order to reduce the possibility of the 'wounded agency', which could counteract well-intended efforts to facilitate a person's recovery.

The various aspects of the medicalisation process that failed to be capability enhancing pointed to 'wounded agency' and the lack of opportunity to assert agency. The language barriers that migrants experienced resulted in difficulties expressing themselves, which did not help build a positive relationship with clinicians. However, where language was not a problem, understanding at the level of meaning, which is important in terms of preserving and building service users' capabilities to be in the driving seat of the recovery journey, was often not facilitated during a medical encounter. 'Wounded agency' could be the result of invalidation. Invalidation does not just happen for service users because discrimination during encounters with the general public. It can happen during encounters with mental health professionals. As Zoie's narrative showed, the pathologisation of her emotional reaction was felt to be a violation of her agency. Carol's sectioning resulted in her changing from being an active seeker for help, to being a 'service avoider'.

The concern about service users' compliance to treatment implies that 'the patient's task is to conform, acquiesce, or yield to the clinician's directives' (Kirmayer, 2001: 26). It contradicts the ethos of the recovery approach, which centrally positions service users' control of their own recovery. Kirmayer proposed that we 'understand patients as actively engaged in understanding their illness and seeking out forms of treatment that make sense to them and fit with salient cultural expectations and social constraints in their lives' (2001: 26). This understanding seems to be important in making sure the process of seeking help is one that contributes to capability enhancement and development.

The interpretive nature of diagnosis opened up a potential gap between medical explanatory models and participants' own understandings of distress (Balint, 1964). Rather than having a fixed presumed set of health beliefs and acting accordingly, participants' explanatory models of their mental distress changed along their recovery journeys. For example, as discussed above, many participants decided to stick to their medication regime not just because of being persuaded by professionals or significant others. They had tried stopping it themselves and got back on to it when they felt that they needed the medicine to maintain a balanced mental state. The pathologisation and medicalisation project is an incomplete one as the co-existence of explanatory models could be found in some participant's narratives.

The variation in participants' experiences can be tracked along the dimensions of migrant/British born, having or not having English language capability and social class. Apart from the economic resources associated with higher-class membership to purchase private health care, social class mattered in the sense that differing class backgrounds of practitioners and service users could impact on the extent that service users were encouraged to be proactive or assert their agency in understanding their ill health and the treatments offered.

The subsequent chapters show how pathologisation and sanism intersect with other dimensions of inequalities in shaping the social conditions participants lived in after acute crisis, and so constitute the different exercisable opportunities the participants have along their recovery journeys.

5 Life after shipwreck

Social conditions for capabilities (re)development

Introduction

This chapter looks at recovery journeys after 'shipwreck', i.e. after a crisis or acute period of mental distress during which participants received medical or psychological intervention. Based on an account of their experiences of using services in rebuilding their lives, it delineates the layers of challenges they encountered when trying to rebuild their lives according to their valued 'being and doing' and analyses which capabilities were (re)developed and which were further diminished.

A main argument of this book is that the social conditions that contribute to distress and ill health in the first place have to be taken into account. Chapter 3 showed how social conditions shaped by inequalities in respect to gender, ethnicity and class contributed to the deprivation and diminishment of participants' capabilities that are important to mental well-being. In this chapter, we will investigate if, and in what way, these lost capabilities were reclaimed or developed and the factors that facilitated and hindered this. Chapter 4 considered the power dimension of the pathologisation process and in what ways different kinds of treatment helped or hindered service users to regain mental well-being. In this chapter, the ways in which persisting symptoms impacted on participants' daily living and building a desired life are considered as well the legacy of the pathologisation process. The experience of power inequality during their encounters with professionals, as well as the ways predicted and perceived risks of future relapse were experienced as a burden and a barrier to seizing life chances will be shown. I argue that these factors were elements of the participants' lived experience that increasingly became shaped by sanism (Chamberlain, 1978; Perlin, 1992; Morrow and Weisser, 2012) and ableism (Parr, 1997; Campbell, 2009), limiting their scope to exercise their agency. This chapter tracks, through participants' narratives, how the ideologies of normalcy and madness, as well as prejudicial assumptions about ability and rationality intersect with social structures in limiting exercisable opportunities for participants.

This chapter is in three sections. The first section considers the assistance and services participants received in rebuilding a life in the community and their perceptions and experiences of these services. Reasons that helped or hindered the participants' capabilities development while using these services will also be analysed. The second section explores whether participants recovered from the capabilities loss that contributed to, or resulted from, their mental ill health. The weight of the structural barriers that are in place as participants try to move on with their lives are illustrated. Structural barriers deprive participants' capabilities to build a life beyond patienthood by limiting their life chances, despite their personal effort in pursuing a flourishing personhood (Barham and Hayward, 1991; Hopper, 2007).

Building a life in the community

Home visits and cultural sensitivity: risk-monitoring or nurturing recovery

Feng, Tang-Yung and Marcus received home visits from nurses, support workers or social workers. Feng had a nurse visit him after his hospital discharge. He felt the service helped him to keep on track with his medication. Tang-Yung and Marcus thought the professionals were more concerned with risk reduction rather than helping them. The medication that Marcus took caused his body to stiffen, which made him immobile at times. He worried about living on his own but felt that the social workers focused on the people he might disturb rather than helping him cope with his difficulties in living, 'Because of my illness, I can't stick to a normal daily routine. I don't cause any damage, I don't want to disturb people. I don't need a social worker to take care of me.'

When Tang-Yung's support worker visited her, Tang-Yung usually asked the Chinese community centre for an interpreter. However, she said there was a time when the support worker filled in a questionnaire without an interpreter present. Tang-Yung disliked the insensitive way that one community nurse asked the 'suicide question'. The nurse asked if she had had thoughts of suicide. Tang-Yung said she did not know what to say, 'She should tell me not to think about suicide, or tell me that there is nothing that can't be solved. It's not good to put it as a question and ask me if I think about suicide.'

What Tang-Yung felt irritated about was that the nurse did not console or counsel her after asking the question. It seemed that the she was looking at Tang-Yung's illness and was concerned with 'risk management', instead of being attentive and talking to her to help alleviate her distress. Again there was no interpreter at this session, so it may have been hard for the nurse to know how to counsel Tang-Yung appropriately.

Interpretation was essential for participants who could not speak English if they were to benefit from a home visit. Such visits had the potential to enable the development of participants' capabilities to live independently and begin to participate in the activities they valued. But the need for practitioners to have the cultural sensitivity to understand subtle cultural meanings embedded in daily practices was important. Tang-Yung described another visit in which a support worker persuaded her to donate the stacks of clothes she did not wear to charity. The worker was probably well intentioned, as this clearance could free up space. But Tang-Yung disliked the worker pressuring her to give up the clothes. It seemed to be experienced by Tang-Yung as disrespecting her agency. She preferred giving the clothes to her friends. Donating clothes to charity and buying second hand might be a common experience for British born people. However, not all migrants are familiar with this practice. Abao, for example, was contemptuous of her in-laws who bought her clothes from charity shops, as she thought it meant that they looked down on her.

Clothes seemed to have a symbolic meaning for Tang-Yung – to her they represented an idea of flourishing that went beyond a lifestyle choice. She held onto her clothes dearly even if they did not fit her anymore. She still had a deep grievance about how the burglary had changed her life course. Chapter 6 considers her attachment to clothes as an adaptive preference she formed after the burglary. She felt she had been trapped in a poor life since. Perhaps the victimhood she embraced meant that she felt she could not afford to give other people a hand. She also hung onto the hope that one day she would wear the clothes again, as she said, 'like the celebrities on the television'. Questions could have been raised, in a sustained exchange between Tang-Yung and her support worker, about whether hanging on to her clothes in this way really contributed to her flourishing. No matter what reasons were behind Tang-Yung's reservation about donating clothes, the meaning behind Tang-Yung's attachment to the clothes might not be easily communicated to a support worker without patience and cultural sensitivity. Such cultural sensitivity is not just about ethnic culture, but in Tang-Yung's narrative is intersected with class and gender.

Supported housing and the quest for independence

Jerry had lived in supported housing since his mental health crisis. Living apart from his parents helped Jerry build his independence. The physical distance gave him space to rebuild his emotional relationship with his parents that he had found difficult to achieve when they were living together. He had been to several mental health placements. At the time of the interview, he lived with ten other service users. Each had their own room while sharing other facilities. The consequence of living in different mental health placements meant that it had been difficult for Jerry to make friends. Although he had a say in where he wanted to live, he felt that there was an element of control in the arrangement.

Author: Why did you have to move?
Jerry: Because of mental health placements. The social worker moved me to this or that hostel or mental health community. There is an element of control here. They control who you are with . . . what types of friends. Also they control what medicines you take and what activities you do.

Jerry thought that the living conditions in the placement were 'very basic'. He did not always get along with other people as he thought many of them had their own serious problems. Sometimes people fought with each other. Jerry experienced racism in the hostel too.

> I had a very big disagreement with somebody in the house I live. He said, 'go back to . . . ' They liked to poke fun or say things like 'you are not British. Go back to China and Hong Kong'. It's not very nice. Not very nice at all. It's horrible.

He told the manager about this. Although the manager consoled him and said 'they talked rubbish', this was still the daily living environment that Jerry had to deal with.

> I can't remember who I said it to. We can't go back to Hong Kong or China because we were born here. I was born here. I can only go back to England. When I go to Hong Kong I go on a British passport. You know. I am a British national. I am a citizen here. You know. The Chinese government won't have us. They won't have us. We have been in this country for a very very long time. We have been here for 40 or 50 years. That's half a life, more than half a life.

Jerry said he would like to get out of the hostel and live independently. I asked what he wanted to do in the future, he said 'I am not wanting a lot of things. I just want my own place (sigh)'.

One of his biggest difficulties, he thought, was that he needed practice cooking his own food. Cooking was not encouraged by the placement, which provided food for the residents. He had to use his own limited benefit money to buy the ingredients if he wanted to cook himself. There was no concrete plan about how to move towards his goal of having his own place. He thought it was all to do with his social worker, who he thought had to help him 'get back into society'. However, they only met once a year. The pace of moving towards his goal was not in his control and he was not assisted in practicing life skills to achieve his goal.

Meeting spaces, information gathering and social activities: the role of statutory services and voluntary organisations for mainstream and Chinese communities

Service users appreciate services that help them gently rebuild day-to-day functioning after a breakdown while providing them with a venue for socialising. Marcus found the NHS rehabilitative services he attended 20 years ago after hospitalisation useful.

Marcus:　Because you gradually . . . it was a like a workshop. It was like you were working, but it was relaxing. Not many days a week, 2 or 3 days. It's like going to work.

Author: A routine?

Marcus: Yes a routine. Those people are experienced. With and without experience is a huge difference. With experience, they are sensitive. Sharp thinking. They know when to push you a bit, but not over stress you.

Apart from being able to pace the redevelopment of his functioning, he valued the opportunities to socialise in the workshop.

> They were quite good in many aspects. First, I am an outgoing person. Second, I can speak English. Third, I am more Westernised in terms of customs. So with the people, they thought I was strange at the beginning. But our distance wasn't that great. I was discriminated against once or twice, but on the whole I had no problem.

Rachel had been attending activities in an NHS day centre in an outpatient clinic for 10 years. Once a week there was a reading or writing group. Rachel explained, 'We write poems. The staff put them in leaflets. I find it quite helpful.'

Rachel was interested in the outings to dance performance as well as visiting galleries and museums. Since she was wary about travelling far unaccompanied, such organised trips were rare chances for her to go to places of interest after her breakdown. However, she said the outpatient clinic had stopped these outings and the writing groups as, she was told, they did not have much funding for these activities. 'It's a shame they change it and stop the group. I think if the group is still on, I would still go to it. There is no group now.'

Voluntary organisations are non-statutory arenas that provided important meeting points for participants to mix with others and engage in social activities. Since the day centre had cut down its activities, a mainstream mental health charity became the only socialising space that Rachel went to regularly, as she only felt comfortable socialising with other service users. She volunteered in a charity shop and allotment every week. Nevertheless, she experienced the effects of changing funding in the charity as well.

> The charity shop has ran out of money. So they are changing. They train people out of work to get back to employment. The mental health volunteers have to 'move on' . . . So, all the volunteers are going and must find new work.

By 'new work', it did not mean that they felt ready to get paid work or, as Rachel had done, seek advice from a job centre about suitable work. The volunteers went separate ways to find volunteering opportunities. Rachel helped out in art classes as an unpaid assistant.

Did the participants who were bilingual speakers prefer mainstream or Chinese voluntary organisations? Young went to a Chinese community centre because his Chinese-speaking parents also participated in the activities and received help. Being able to offer a family-oriented approach is one of the main strengths of

Chinese community centres – they could cater for the different language needs across different generations within a family. This approach could develop service users' capability to maintain the family relations they valued. Marcus was critical of some 'Chinese customs'. However, his social worker referred him to a Chinese community centre. He felt that the social worker did not know how to deal with him and assumed what he needed was contact with other Chinese people.

> You can say it was discrimination or wearing a coloured lens. He doesn't know how to deal with you, because of your different customs. So he hoped the Chinese association could help. But I am used to the way of expressing things in English in the UK.

Marcus' experience of being 'pigeonholed' illustrated the importance of understanding cultural practices as fluid. Failing to do so, service providers ran the risk of mistaking stereotypical 'culturalist' assumptions for 'cultural sensitivity'. For participants who could not speak fluent English, the role of Chinese community centres or Chinese church's help was paramount.

Providing information about benefits and available services is an important function of voluntary organisations. Participants who knew little about benefits and support said it was often through personal networks and the outreach of community centres that they gained knowledge.

Abao had not known that Carer's Allowance existed during the 20 years she had been her husband's carer until she had a breakdown and was helped by a Chinese community centre. In fact, apart from Income Support, she and her husband was not aware that they could apply for disability benefits even though her husband had been to the doctors requesting proof of his learning difficulties. It was through the Chinese community centre that an arrangement was set up for her to properly assess the household's needs. While Abao's experience indicated that there had been a lack of care from statutory services, Jerry said that he felt there was, in his words, 'an element of control', because of his extensive and long involvement in the services. Jerry, through volunteering in a Chinese centre, kept abreast of the changes of legislation regarding rights in relation to mental health and other areas. He felt that knowledge about rights and entitlements was important to retaining self-determination and independence.

Jerry: I worry about things like law ... It's the English law I have to deal with.
Author: What do you mean 'you have to deal with'?
Jerry: Like benefits. That's law. Inheritance, if you know ... If eventually my parents ...
Author: You mean you have to know your rights.
Jerry: Yes. You have to know your rights and what you are entitled to. What else is there? Mental health law. What the doctor can do and say. What they can't do and say. If I have a place of my own one day ... that's all law basically. Your finance. What coming in and what's going out.

Opportunities for socialising in Chinese community centres and Chinese churches were appreciated by some participants. It is clear that community development in terms of fostering the growth and sustainability of non-government organisations is crucial in developing the capabilities of community members. Ken thought that his worldview was more akin to Buddhism than Christianity, but he considered being able to join in Church activities was important to his recovery. Volunteering helped Lai-Ming to feel that he had 'improved' from being someone who received help from others to someone who offered help to others. The programmes run by Chinese community centres about mental health, such as a service user-run café bar and befriending programme, seemed to enable some participants to see community centres as trusted sources of help as well as a means of building their connectedness with other service users.

Connectedness is considered important in the recovery literature (e.g. Ware *et al.*, 2007; Weisser *et al.*, 2011; Slade *et al.*, 2012; Tew *et al.*, 2012). In what way can connectedness contribute to capability development? Ware *et al.* (2007) detailed what connectedness means. The three elements they identified are useful in evaluating the quality of connectedness to make it become a capability, i.e. how social networks can become social capital that can be utilised (Portes, 1998). They can also explain barriers towards building connectedness, i.e. how some participants felt wary of extending their social networks.

Connectedness involves a maintenance of reciprocal interpersonal relationships (Ware *et al.*, 2007). Carol found housework and caring for her child stressful while having to cope with her fluctuating symptoms. However, she was reluctant to ask friends to help as she did not feel able to return the favour because of the unpredictability of the distress she experienced every day. Also, reciprocity entailed a code of cultural practice that was understood and adopted by both sides. With the heterogeneity within the Chinese communities, in respect to place of origin, dialects and regional ethnic groups, misunderstandings of cultural practice can be a barrier to forming relationships. Marcus saw himself as 'Westernised' and called the code of cultural practice 'an interaction problem' in the Chinese community centre.

Marcus: The way the Chinese express things are different. Like if I say I don't have money I don't want to go out today, they would be puzzled, thinking whether I am asking them for money.

Author: Like hinting something, but actually you are just simply saying you don't want to go out?

Marcus: Yes. Not wanting to go out just means not wanting to go out. But some people would think they have upset you so you want to avoid them. This is irritating.

This also explained the burden Shun-Tien felt in socialising.

Sometimes when you talk too much you may say something wrong that makes other people unhappy. Many of them speak a different dialect from me. If I say something wrong they may tell others. It's troublesome. I don't want trouble.

The 'trouble' Shun-Tien anticipated was fear of gossip. Gossip and worrying about being talked about behind one's back hindered the development of trust in relationships. Trust is another way to understand reciprocity in personal relationships.

The second element of connectedness is social currency, which refers to personal characteristics such as talents, demeanor and physical attractiveness. Such social currencies are about how individuals befriend some people but not others (Ware *et al.*, 2007). One participant who joined the befriending programme had another user visit her home and vice versa. Although she was polite and did not show her dislike of the visitor, she did not feel that a friendship had been formed and did not really want her to visit too often.

Although befriending might be a way to create opportunities for reciprocity, it might not necessarily develop into long-term friendships. Ware *et al.*'s (2007) third element was 'identifying with a larger group' and referred to the subjective sense of belonging to a group perceived to have something in common. Such a sense of belonging could be related to an individual's identification with an ethnic group but it also means much more than that. This entails service users moving on beyond the arena of community when they want to, and expanding their social roles to pursue their valued being and doing beyond patienthood. Did social conditions enable or disable participants to do this? What were the ordeals they endured along the journey?

Recovering from social conditions or further capability deprivation

'Go home'? Belonging, citizenship and positionality

'Go home' is a common racist phrase encountered by ethnic minorities. Racism can prevent service users develop supporting and understanding relationships with each other. Although Jerry was born in Britain and lived with his family in the UK, he had been told to 'go back to your own country' by other service users in his mental health placement as shown above. Migrants like overseas brides, who thought that not getting used to life in the UK life was a source of their distress, wanted to go home but could not. Going home as a way of regaining capabilities from their adjustment problems was not always a feasible choice. Over time their links with relatives in their home country could be weakened.

For example, Nin-Jin's husband had passed away and her children were all grown up. Although she was free from domestic responsibilities, she preferred to stay in the UK with her children and bear those aspects of UK life that she did not like. Tang-Yung had lost trust in her family in mainland China who had forced her to go into a psychiatric hospital. She did not want to go back to her home country to avoid contact with her family.

For many participants, economic reasons were another factor for not being able to migrate back to their home country. Most participants who came to the UK through marriage were not economically independent. Carol had explored the possibility of going back to Hong Kong after her breakdown in the UK. For the first few years after her post-natal depression, she spent half the year in the UK and half in Hong Kong, where she had parental family support to take care of her and help out with the baby. Although possessing dual nationalities allowed her to keep a foot in both countries, moving back and forth was not viable in the long term. At one point she considered leaving her husband and staying in Hong Kong. She asked a Hong Kong social worker about the benefits she could apply for and explored work options. However, she was given a 'lecture'.

> The social workers are on the same floor as the doctor. Their departments are right next to each other. There was one social worker. Male. I remember this guy very well. I really wanted to beat him up. We talked face to face. I said I wanted a divorce. I didn't want to keep dragging my husband down. He shouted at me, you know! 'What qualifications have you got? You only graduated from junior secondary school. What is the qualification of your husband? University graduate! You would abandon him? No one will want you if you try to get a job now! You are fat and ugly.' He really pointed at me and lectured me! Fuck! I really want to beat him up! (Chuckle) I didn't. Why? If I do, I will be in great trouble. Because right away you can be taken away by the doctor and staff to the psychiatric unit next door. Dare not dream to get out. So I have to put up with him, you know. How hard it was to put up with him in the room! There wasn't a single sentence that wasn't insulting. Not one sentence that didn't lecture me! I didn't say a word. I could only cry on the way.

This insulting and discriminating 'lecture' came from her allegedly 'own' people in Hong Kong. Sadly, what the social worker said about limited job opportunities for middle-aged women with low educational qualifications was not far from the truth in the Hong Kong labour market. However, in light of the disadvantage in the labour market Carol might face, the apparently patronising and prejudiced attitude of the social worker in this case discouraged and disadvantaged Carol from exploring and accessing possible support services that might have helped Carol to return to Hong Kong. What Carol eventually chose to do is not the most important concern in a Capabilities analysis based on a structural approach of recovery. What is important is that Carol was not informed of available options and supports. She was at the stage of seeking information and she might very well have decided to stay in the UK anyway. However, the prejudice from the social worker she experienced was demoralising and invalidated her agency as a woman seeking independence.

Going home was also not an option for Feng. As mentioned in Chapter 3, it was difficult for him and his wife to earn enough money to repay the debt that they owed the snakehead for smuggling them into the UK. During his hospitalisation, his wife succeeded in applying for legal residency status for the family. Apart from the economic considerations, Feng considered that staying in the UK provided him with the recovery space he needed.

> This kind of thing (mental illness) does not mean you can recover just by
> going back to China. I don't understand . . . I don't understand what kind of
> illness I have. I don't know very well. But I know for sure that I have an ill-
> ness. I am totally different from normal people.

Going back home is not the same as returning to a familiar environment. For
Feng, the home country had become a new environment after his absence and
life-changing events like a mental breakdown. A new environment could pose
new challenges. Feng thought it was important to take his process of recovery
slowly.

> Giving myself too big a challenge is not good. It's not good. It's better to
> take it slowly. Slowly adjust to the environment. Slowly to see how to change
> myself. Adjust my psychological state, slowly. For example, you can't say
> everyone who gets this psychological illness overseas would definitely get
> better if they go home. I can't say for sure going home is the best for me.
> It depends on how severe you are and what treatment you need. If it's not
> severe, if your thinking is still ok, you can try new environments, going back
> home. Not a big challenge or sudden change, but take it slowly. If you jump
> back home, for certain you can't take it.

His legal status to remain in the UK meant that his capabilities for a decent living
were expanded as he was now entitled to statutory health and social services and
benefit, which were important conversion factors that enabled him to redevelop
daily functioning. It allowed him a space of recovery that he felt he needed and
was important after his hospitalisation. He was unsure about whether he would
like to stay in the UK in the long run. However, his UK legal status gave him the
capability to choose to go back to mainland China in the future. He did not have
to live in the corner of UK society or at the margins of his home country when he
was still trying to regain his daily functioning. His legal status stopped a chain of
capabilities loss.

The stories of Nin-Jin, Tang-Yung, Carol and Feng warned against roman-
ticising the notion of going home. Hins found that coming to the UK allowed
her to distance herself from stigma in her hometown. Her story also illustrated
that the so-called traditional Chinese values of close-knit kinship networks, like
other cultural practices, were fluid in the sense that members of the culture could
choose to embrace them or not. Hins was the only participant who felt sure that
she would not have another relapse. Despite her confidence that her mental
health illness was a thing of the past, other people kept reminding her about
it. Hins found it difficult to assert survivorship in her home kinship network in
China. Coming to the UK to pursue postgraduate study not only expanded her
capabilities to develop a career, it also widened her capabilities to deal with
mental health prejudice by enabling her to distance herself from close relatives
and family members who saw her as a mental patient, instead of a survivor over-
coming setbacks in life.

My mom told relatives about my past. She said, 'you see my girl. My girl survived it'. They still say my illness was not recovered. But my mom said, 'You see, with all the hardship who else can overcome it? Yet we are fine'.

Hins and her mother tried to assert a narrative of survivorship in their close-knit family circle. This strong tie became a source of stress for Hins.

Author: Why did they say you haven't recovered?
Hins: Because my life trajectory was different from other people. For others, lives are smooth. Like you don't have to put a great deal of care and effort and you went through it. But me . . .
Author: You mean they thought it was because of your illness that your lives weren't smooth. But actually it was other factors (Hins had been recounting her other setbacks in life apart from her mental health crisis).
Hins: Yes. External factors. That's why they talked like that and made assumptions. I didn't want to stay in that circle.

Hins stressed how she had built her own life – personhood from patienthood (Barham and Hayward, 1991). She had been working hard to develop her career and had not had a relapse since her childhood. She was not on long-term medication and was confident she would not have a relapse. However, her immediate family-community would often remind her of her past. Such stereotyping and discrimination prevented her building an identity beyond patienthood, despite her effort and hard work. She disliked the way her relatives thought she was abnormal, as if they had put an indelible stamp on her.

> For many years I have had success, like my career. They can see that. But I always have this feeling that they are talking about me behind my back, as they knew my past very well. Although they are my relatives and want me to be fine, I wonder if they see me with their memory of my past. Because I think I am a very normal person, aren't I? No matter how big the setbacks I encountered I survived them. I didn't want them to see me in that way again.

I asked if this stigma had anything to do with her coming to the UK. She said yes. Hins described her perception of stigma in mainland China.

> In the mainland China, people liked to see you with 'coloured glasses'. Like the old Chinese saying, 'once you are bitten by a snake, you would be scared of it forever'. It's like once you had this history . . . I don't like this. Because a person can have a new life. Also it was not my fault to have this history. It was those . . . I think I was unlucky. All the bad things happened to me. If those kids had not done horrible things to me, I wouldn't have developed this in my personality. I mean I felt that the impact of the bullying goes with me all the time. Even now. I tend to get defensive, unlike other people who are compliant.

Coming to the UK helped maintain a distance from her kinship circle, which increased her capability to engage with, or be free from them, in a way she wanted. She was very careful not to reveal her mental health history to her new friends in the UK, so she could build a new identity.

These different narratives illuminated the complex ways belonging is experienced (Anthias, 2006). They counter the 'go home' discourse, which assumes ethnic minorities are welcomed by the geographical space called the 'home country'. The construction of home country out of an imagined belonging glosses over the inequalities of capabilities within the home country. Inequalities of gender and social class, as in Carol's situation, Feng's uncertain project of 're-inclusion' into his home country and the prejudiced judgement Hins experienced in her kinship network were exclusionary forces located in home countries, which created obstacles to capabilities development towards independence, favourable inclusion and personhood (Sen, 2000)

Unpaid and paid caring work, self-worth and economic empowerment

Building a life for oneself was a theme in the recovery journey of full-time carers. Counselling gave Abao a space to vent her stress. Bai-Xin thought that she had to change her entire life and tell herself to be happy. She took control her daily life, keeping a regular routine to exercise in the park every morning, playing music at home while doing housework, and going out to window shop when the pressure from her husband became too much to handle. She also joined activities organised for carers in the Chinese community centres whenever possible. Carers taking care of themselves increased the capability of the cared for as well. As Bai-Xin put it,

> My husband is a patient himself. He can't give me happiness. What can you do? Even if he doesn't give me space, I still have to be happy. If he doesn't accommodate me and I collapse because of that, it is bad. Gradually he would get ill; I would get ill. This situation is what I dislike most.

Her psychological work, self-care and caring activities were still demanding and not easy to share with other people. Abao's husband only felt safe with her and liked to follow her around. She wanted a holiday to visit her family in China, but hiring a carer for her husband was difficult as he was reluctant to socialise with other people. She was not sure if her friends would be willing to care for her husband for a short period on a paid basis.

Her narrative conveyed the weight of caring as gendered work. Patriarchy devalues caring and housework (DeVault, 1994). Yet, the stress Carol faced in her recovery journey revealed how taking care of the family was a laborious task. She was a full-time housewife.

> My husband says I have done an excellent job. Why? Antidepressants make you very tired. Because it aims to cool you down. You are then given tranquillisers on

top of it. The tranquillisers make you even more tired. And then you add sleeping pills. Wouldn't you become so tired that you sleep like a pig? But I can only sleep 4 to 5 hours a day. I have a lot of pressure.

The pressure is not tangible. Like now it's 2 o'clock. I have to tell myself to prepare a sandwich later for my son to eat after school. I have to go out shopping because there is not enough food for dinner. The pressure as a housewife is tremendous.

Carol described how her fluctuating mental state was like a relapse. I asked what she meant by relapse. She elaborated vividly on the pressure of having to cope with fluctuating distress and changing symptoms.

Relapse means that day I will cry. My temper will be strange. I won't care to respond to you. If you say anything, I will shout at you but I won't know what I shout about. Some memories will be lost. This is my situation right now. My obsession disorder is quite severe. It becomes obsession disorder right now. If the dishes are not washed after a meal, I will be very agitated and can't help cleaning them all up. Once they are cleaned I will be very relieved. The clothes have to be cleaned every week. If there is a tiny bit of dirt somewhere, it becomes an eyesore to me . . . A lot of things . . . when you have a relapse, you don't have a clear mind. But you would still stand in the kitchen finishing all the stuff. The next day I would wonder why my arms were so tired. I would try to recall anything I had done.

Doing housework this way can be dangerous. Carol told herself, 'I can't carry on like this'. I have to keep myself awake so as to cook the meal. Otherwise accidents can happen.

Because of her fluctuating and unpredictable symptoms, she was reluctant to ask friends to help with household chores or take her son home from school as she thought she would not be able to reciprocate.

Abao, Bai-Xin, Carol and other overseas brides said that their children were their source of satisfaction. Nevertheless, self-realisation outside domesticity was something that they tried to seek. Abao wanted to look for work although she had been stopped from this by her in-laws in the past. Carol also expressed her hope to work. While Wu-Wei took pride in her children, she said her paid work gave her the most satisfaction. She used her caring skills to work in a home for the elderly.

I feel that working with the elderly makes me feel that I am a useful person. I feel a sense of satisfaction that I can help others while earning money. Working makes me feel that I can contribute to society. I want to prove that I am a useful person.

In recovering from the shame that resulted from the hidden injuries of class and gender (discussed in Chapter 3), paid work helped improve her self-image.

Although the money she earned was not enough for economic independence, it contributed to her economic empowerment (Aydinligil, 2009). She saved her salary for herself. This meant that she had her own money and eased her sense of insecurity about the future.

Setting up home with her husband away from her in-laws had given her a sense of relief. She did not have to worry about taking orders from her in-laws and could arrange her home to her own liking. It had not been not easy for her to stray away from the 'Chinese tradition'.

> I didn't dare. My husband and I discussed setting up own home, but I didn't dare. My grandmother in mainland China kept telling me to live with my in-laws till they die. To take care of them till they die. Our Chinese tradition . . . I came to the UK to live with them. Now living away from the parents-in-law, I am free. When I go home, I feel so free. This is my home. I can do whatever I want. I can tidy when I want. Most importantly is that I don't feel pressure from in-laws. I don't feel coming home is a burden anymore.

Barriers in the labour market

Wu-Wei's experience seems to confirm the argument of Sen (1997) and Leff and Warner (2006) that employment can facilitate recovery in terms of validating one's worth as well as providing material resources. However, as discussed in Chapter 3, it can be a source of stress that diminishes an individual's capability to benefit from employment. What enabled employment to be capability enhancing for Wu-Wei seems to relate to the sector she worked in. Her employer knew about her last breakdown. She worried about losing the job.

> They insisted on visiting me even though my husband rejected them. After that they asked the doctor . . . they waited for a long time . . . I already assumed that I would lose the job. They might worry that I would hurt the elderly. So I didn't want to go back. They asked the doctor to write a letter stating that I wasn't violent. They let me go back to work after receiving the letter. Also I found a job in a fast-food chain at that time. They saw they I had the ability to work there and take care of my children. So they hired me again. I have worked with the elderly for many years, we developed a good relationship.

The willingness of her employer to take her back was perhaps because of the non-profit nature of the sector she worked for. It could be also because it was difficult to find another worker to replace her as she had already developed relationships with the elderly people she cared for. She was relatively protected compared to other participants looking for jobs in for-profit market.

Chapter 3 showed that the work environment, especially the harsh working conditions in Chinese catering resulted in the deprivation of mental well-being for some participants. They were also pessimistic about their chances in the mainstream labour market because of perceived racial discrimination. Some participants were not in work at the time of their breakdown. Those who had to leave university because of a breakdown tried to look for employment. Their loss of capabilities to find employment because of their period of ill health was difficult to recover from, as they faced further disadvantages resulting from mental health discrimination.

Many participants avoided Chinese catering work in which they had previously fallen ill. To remain flexible, to accommodate the fluctuation of his symptoms, Marcus looked for freelance jobs via his friends. Lai-Ming, Ken and Young went to job centres to look for job openings. It was difficult to gain a foothold in the mainstream labour market. All the participants faced the burden of whether to disclose their history of mental health problems or not (Wheat *et al.*, 2010). Marcus was very cautious when telling me his diagnosis. We held the interview in a 'Western' chain café in Chinatown. He looked around and then wrote down 'paranoid schizophrenia' in my notebook. Marcus relied on his friendship network for freelance work so he felt he had to hide his diagnosis.

In contrast, Young, Lai-Ming and Ken thought that they had to disclose their mental health history to potential employers. Young could not hide his history because the workplace required him to get a letter from a doctor to say he was fit for work. Ken thought hiding his mental health conditions would give him trouble after reading a court case (*Cheltenham Borough Council v Laird*) in which a council sued its former managing director for withholding her history of depression (BBC, 15 June 2009). Although the council lost the case, the message Ken took from it was not a reassuring one. He was unaware that he could be protected under the then Disability Discrimination Act by choosing non-disclosure. The possibility that one could be sued for non-disclosure and the grueling legal procedures that followed was enough for Ken to feel that he did not have a choice to withhold his mental health history. A gap in his CV because of the period of breakdown and ill health was a concern. Lai-Ming thought that even if you did not disclose, employers would ask you about gaps in your CV. Ken did not know what to put down on his CV because of the break that he took to slowly rebuild his life. A full-time uninterrupted career path in the labour market is a socially constructed norm that excludes people with gaps in their CV as a result of disability, illness or domestic commitment (Arun *et al.*, 2004).

Work opportunities were further reduced because of ethnic inequalities and ageism. Lai-Ming who was over 60 had only managed to get two jobs since his breakdown in his early twenties. Both jobs did not last for long. Lai-Ming thought racial and disability discrimination prevented him from securing jobs after interviews: 'First, we have "yellow face". They don't want foreigners. Discrimination. Racial discrimination. Compared to other interviewees, our marks will be deducted. Second, you had nervous breakdown. They would hire someone normal'.

Despite these hurdles, Lai-Ming kept going to job centres and attending sessions with disability officers, even though he thought that both he and the disability officer knew that he would not be able to get a job at his age. Ageism further increased the disadvantages participants experienced in the labour market. Participants who had breakdowns in middle age, or mental health difficulties that persisted into their middle years faced ageism. Job seeking was considered by Ken as one of the barriers on his recovery journey. Comparing the job markets in the UK and Hong Kong, Ken thought that it would be easier for him to find a job in the UK. 'Here in the UK it is more realistic to get a job . . . In Hong Kong what can you do? Maybe a fast-food restaurant. It is difficult to find work in Hong Kong when you are middle aged.'

Ken was in his mid-forties at the time of the interview. He had worked in the UK information technology (IT) sector for many years and had worked in various jobs including teaching in a secondary school and university in Hong Kong. His pessimism about not being able to find jobs in similar fields again reflected his observation about age discrimination in Hong Kong. It also reflected how biography interlinks with social change. Having left the IT sector for other jobs, followed by a period of rest during and after his mental health crisis, he did not think his IT experience, knowledge and skills were relevant anymore given the rapid development in the sector. He experienced deskilling.

> I can't return to the past. I could not work in IT any more because there are so many technological advances to catch up with. Age is a big concern. To be honest, I don't think people would hire me in IT even if I tried.

He considered openness and diversity as a key factor in deciding where he might rebuild a working life.

> I think there is more diversity in terms of jobs here (the UK). I can try different types of work. That's how I feel. Hong Kong is more rigid. If you had worked in the information technology field, it is not easy for you to change path.

Ken went to job centres to look for job openings. In fact, he was interviewed for a job in IT, which, he later realised, required him to put money into training before being officially employed. He had not yet found a job at the time of interview. It seems that the UK labour market was not as diverse and open as he hoped.

Challenges in keeping a job and a chain of capabilities loss

When participants got a job in the mainstream labour market, keeping it was a challenge. Because of their lack of educational qualifications, the 'Western jobs' they could get were low-skilled manual jobs with poor working conditions. In the experiences of Lai-Ming and Young, there was a chain of capabilities loss.

Lai-Ming found a job in a printing factory after hospitalisation from his first breakdown. He was in charge of operating the printing machine. The machine was very noisy, making it difficult for him to concentrate.

The machine was very noisy. It was very noisy in the working areas. You needed high concentration when operating it. Slight deviation will ruin the printing. It's very noisy. You hear the buzzing sounds. It's like someone keeps shouting "weeeeeeeeeee" to your ears. Later on my ear problem developed and I could not balance myself when standing next to it.

The workplace did not provide him with earplugs or other occupational safety equipment. After a year he had to see the doctor for his ear problem. After taking a few days of leave from work because of the problem, he got a note from his boss telling him not to come back to work again. Since then, in his words, he 'joined the army of the unemployed'. This happened 30 years ago when he was in his early thirties. He never hid his disability status from his employers and kept going to the job centre to look for jobs, seeing disability officers there. However, he was not been able to find a full-time or stable part-time job again.

Unemployment does not only mean a loss of secure income. It brings other capabilities loss (Sen, 1997). Being unemployed is dispiriting, it has a negative impact on a person's self-worth. During the interview, Lai-Ming went to great lengths to explain the details of his printing job and said he was proud of himself for knowing how to operate the machine. Being out of work took away this sense of pride. His words illustrated the psychological harm of the unemployment as a result of ableism. 'If you are not disabled you are then abled. I can work. After the nervous breakdown, sometimes I would feel sad. A sense of loss. I have to have medicine to help me. Friends helped me too.' His sense of loss reflects how his recovery journey was hampered by poor working conditions and unemployment. His words also reflect how he felt about 'disability' – the line marking 'who is fit to work' restricts people's participation in employment, depriving people of opportunities to develop skills, mastery and autonomy as well as contribute to society. Ableism is a negative social conversion factor, which rendered the opportunity gradient of Lai-Ming's life chances shallow.

Young had worked in a few different jobs for short periods. He said it was his mental illness that was part of the reason that he quit and found another job. The other reason for working on a short-term basis was because he could only find jobs on short-term contracts. Young disclosed his psychiatric diagnosis to employers because they wanted proof of his fitness to work. The consequences of disclosure were negative.

Young: I think . . . maybe it affected how other people think of me. At work if people know I have this kind of illness, there may be disturbance . . . They said I did things wrong. They said I made mistakes. I felt they didn't welcome me to work there.

Author: What did you do when they said that?

Young: I usually negotiated with them. Negotiate with the boss, or the manager. I explained how I can work better.

Work was a terrain in which Young felt he had to fight constantly to defend himself. Although he felt he was being treated unfairly, he could not be sure. There were times when he thought he was not the only one who made mistakes or was slow, and his colleagues were being unfair to him. He recalled his experience in his last job in a laboratory.

Young: Yes I did feel they were unfair to me. But the boss couldn't oversee everything. So it was down to how I explained the situation. If I could explain myself, then he could let me to carry on working; if not, then he would tell me to see a doctor, or send me to do other stuff.
Author: Do you feel able to assert yourself?
Young: Half and half. I am not that good.

The situation in which he was accused of slow working was related to his persisting symptoms:

> When I was ill, I had headaches and I felt my body can't move. I would want to rest. My whole body . . . I felt like it was stopped. Even if I was working, I had to stop and rest for a while and then carry on. When I see things, I have to rest and sleep. They felt real. And I felt like what happened around me had stopped. When they clear away, I can become myself again. Without seeing things, I can be myself and carry on working. If it happens when I am on the street, I slow down and try to think clearly.

When the symptoms struck at work, he would not know how long he had stopped working. Some colleagues would say he had stopped for an hour. Some said 3 hours. He didn't know who to believe.

Young: Sometimes I think they worked less than me. They forced me to work more than the others. If I worked less than them, they might tell me off, saying that I worked too slow.
Author: Did you reflect this to your boss?
Young: He reacted by apology.
Author: You mean they apologised?
Young: I mean they accepted my apology.
Author: Why was it you who apologised?
Young: There was no other way.
Author: So you apologised for working slowly, even though on some occasions you felt that you were picked on by the colleagues?
Young: Yes.

I asked if he had ever requested a third-party representative, for example, from a trade union, to assess if his work performance was down to his illness or he was being unfairly treated. He didn't know how to approach the trade union and thought that the trade union would not solve the problem. From what he observed in one of his past workplaces, he thought the trade union would not act on a work-er's behalf unless a strong case was put together. As he was not confident that he could put forward a strong case about his work performance, he felt he could only rely on himself. I asked if his employer made any reasonable adjustment for him as he declared himself disabled before starting the job.

Young: They consider the business, not my health. They won't accommodate
me. They consider the business and think what work they need people
to do and find the appropriate person to do it. If I am not suitable for the
job, they will ask me to leave.
Author: So when you felt ill at work, they wouldn't give you any support?
Young: They wouldn't. They only told me to get well soon. They said other-wise I would lose my job.

Eventually he was told he didn't work well and was fired. 'They didn't say it was related to my illness. They said I was lazy. They just look at the business. The profit. They didn't consider whether I had illness or not.'

Declaring disability at the point of employment seemed to strengthen the employer's control over workers, in this case, instead of protecting Young from disadvantage and discrimination. Since being fired from this job, he had been unemployed for 5 years. When I interviewed him he was looking for jobs but was demoralised because of his unemployment. Young's situation had resulted in loss of skill, which is capability diminishing (Sen, 1997). He was worried that he would not be able to work again because he had been out of work for so long. Although he was doing volunteer work at the Chinese com-munity centre, he felt that he was out of touch with the real working world. 'It's like something is lacking. It's like I am never able to get something done or achieve anything.'

In contrast to Lai-Ming and Young who could find 'Western' jobs because of their English language skills, Feng could only go back to Chinese catering. As explored in Chapter 3, it was a sector in which workers lacked bargaining power. Compared to Young who tried to negotiate with his employer, Feng hid his psy-chiatric diagnosis from his boss and used self-exclusion as a strategy to protect himself. Feng felt sure that he could only manage part-time work. He thought that his persisting symptoms or the side effects of medication interfered with his work as a kitchen helper. I asked which aspects of the work he found difficult. It turned out that it was the stigmatising and bullying environment, rather than coping with the symptoms. He worked part-time to avoid interacting with other workers.

I don't have problem doing the work. Just that . . . if I work for a long time, other workers would chat and I could only react slowly. My reaction is slow. Dumb. The boss and other people would become suspicious, thinking 'oh, does this guy have mental illness?' In such working environments conflict is common. Then your thinking will become unhealthy again. Psychological illness will emerge again. Then I do not want to work. I want to escape. I will then isolate myself. Lock myself up. So when I work part-time, I work only two days. I am ok when my hands are full, busily working. I have no problem working. You got busy for two days. When time is up, you go home. The boss won't be able to find out (about his mental illness) when I am busy working two days.

In the harsh working conditions of Chinese catering it is highly unlikely that disability discrimination legislation and the concept of reasonable adjustment had ever taken root. This means it was up to workers to resort to self-limiting and individualised strategies to deal with potential discrimination. Feng was able to fulfill the tasks required of him as a worker in the restaurant. It was not exhaustion from this physical work that kept him from working more hours. Working part-time was a way he used to gauge his steps in getting back to employment. For Feng, part of his capabilities loss was the lowering of self-esteem. The unfavorable work conditions seemed to hinder the development of this capability, which was crucial for his participation in the community.

> I am really scared that people will look down on me. But this is how everyone would normally react. However . . . first of all you have to know that you have this psychological illness. You can misunderstand people . . . misunderstand how other people think of you. First, don't take this . . . don't take what people say about you to your heart. People's reactions [stigma] are normal. Most importantly it's whether you can let it pass. Because you've got this psychological illness. I mean . . . I've got this illness, I have to . . . have to console myself. I got this illness . . . I have to take medications, treatment. To recover, etc.
>
> You can't say . . . 'Oh this person talks about me behind my back'. First you need to understand yourself. Understand to what degree your psychological state has recovered. Everyone has psychological illness. But . . . how should I say . . . Although people say everyone has psychological illness, some have enough will power to withstand it. Some people do not have enough will power. If you don't have enough will power, when you encounter a sudden setback or being shocked, your reaction would be abnormal. So you have to sober up. You have to improve yourself. You have to change psychologically. This will help you recover.
>
> I think right now the degree of my recovery . . . my thought is still . . . abnormal. Chatting or like doing an interview, I can do it. But I think my thinking . . . is not healthy enough. My psychological reaction is not healthy enough.

The paranoia and voice-hearing that Feng experienced during his crisis reduced his confidence about socialising with people. The adverse working conditions in catering were unhelpful in rebuilding his confidence in this area too. Instead of thinking it could be other people's reactions to him that contributed to this situation, he saw it as his problem due to his symptoms and that it was up to him to manage. He took on an illness identity to self-manage perceived stigma and rationalise other people's behaviour as normal and his worry about stigma as abnormal. The way Feng took on his illness identity and considered his avoidance of socialising as 'lacking willpower' was capability diminishing. This illustrated the problematic of illness identity – self-identification as mentally ill has a negative impact on one's hope and self-esteem (Yanos *et al.*, 2010). In Feng's experience, while mental ill health did not interfere with his performance at work, his feelings of incompetence constrained his capabilities for social connectedness.

Measures that aimed to increase the employability of service users were not very useful in Young, Rachel and Raymond's experience. They had had job coaching and received on the spot training as sales assistants in a chain department store or doing errands for the local authority. However, the message they got was that there were not many jobs around and not everyone could get a job after completing the programme.

The benefit system and discourse: safety net, conversion factors and the disciplining effect

Because of the barriers in the labour market and prolonged unemployment, benefits were essential to many participants' survival. In relation to capabilities development, benefits acted as a safety net for the household, which stopped capabilities deprivation. Feng thought benefits were enough to provide the basics for his family of four, while Nin-Jin thought they provided just about enough for her family if she watched her budget carefully. Carers' allowance served as a financial subsidy for the whole household when carers could not take on paid work because of their full-time caring tasks. Bai-Xin used some of her allowance to buy herself clothes 'as a treat' to relieve her stress from caring and take care of herself.

While benefits provided some participants with a safety net the operation of the benefit system and discourses about benefits acted as a negative conversion factor that prevented recipients develop further capabilities. Rachel was very wary of getting paid work, as she was told her benefits would be affected. It felt like the rug had been pulled from under her feet.

Rachel: Because as long as I'm on benefit, I can always go to the psychiatrist, if I feel unwell mentally. And if I have any relapse or any concerns about my progress, I can always go to the doctors. But if I get into a job, they . . . It would just take a long long time to get back into the system.
Author: Do you mean that if they sign a letter saying you are fit to work, they will cut you off from the services?
Rachel: Yes. And then I will take a long time to get back into the system again.

She raised similar concerns about going back to university. The way benefits acted as a safety net was not experienced by Rachel as capability enabling. It was not, as 'welfare to work' proponents argue, that the existence of a benefit safety net discouraged participants from getting a job. For Rachel it was the perceived obstacles that she might encounter in going into work and the vulnerability she felt that discouraged her from moving into paid employment. This feeling of vulnerability is not an individual deficiency but a result of a realistic assessment of labour market barriers.

The disciplining effect of the benefit scroungers discourse was reflected in the narratives of Ken, Feng and Lai-Ming. Ken was eligible to apply for disability living allowance (DLA) but he did not apply for it. He was relying on his savings, which were likely to run out shortly. The reason he did not apply for DLA was that he did not consider himself 'very disabled'. Also the church told him that getting benefits might make him lose his dignity, which would make him feel worse. For Feng and Lai-Ming, this discourse reinforced the abnormal and disabled identities they had taken on to protect themselves from criticism. Feng felt he had to justify the benefits he received,

> I am not greedy for government's welfare. Some people are normal, more normal than me. They just take the welfare and do not want to work. Lazy bones. I am different. Because I have psychological illness, I cannot work. But I want to be a normal people and accept the normal work environment.

In Lai-Ming's view,

> I always admit that I have a disability. I know it. I have actually been in hospital. I was on benefit. I was on medical treatment and I did not cheat the government for money. The hundred something quid benefits, the pension credit . . . You lost your ability to work and the low pay you got. That's why they give you the money. I am not those who cheat. Those who lie about their sickness. Like those Black women who gave birth to ten or more children and the children just took the benefits instead of taking a job.

These interview extracts show how dominant benefit discourses encourage discrimination against other ethnic minorities and have a disciplinary effect that is disempowering and restricts the exercise of agency. Lai-Ming was clear that he had to prove that he was not lazy.

Lai-Ming: I know that when I did the waiter job, I sometimes broke stuff. If they didn't sack me I would sack myself. I only worked for a few days. But even just for a few days, I can show it to the government. See? I worked. I had paid tax.

Author: Why is that important?

Lai-Ming: Why? When people ask you when you claim the pension, 'why hadn't you paid tax for a long time?' . . . If I had even a few days of work history, I can prove that it's not that I didn't want to work. It's not that I am lazy. Not that I am greedy for your benefit and did not want to

work. Of course I want to earn money. Benefit is not enough . . . So
when people asked me why I took government's money all the time,
I could say I had looked for jobs but just that people didn't hire me.

Conclusions

If there was a common theme across the recovery journeys of the participants,
it is that they were striving to get back into the driving seat of their lives. In
this chapter, I have shown what helped the participants rebuild a life according
to their valued 'being and doing' and what hindered their efforts. This chapter
has focused on the community level and explored the ways community services had positive and negative impacts on the social inclusion experienced by
participants. The cultural sensitivity of staff was shown to be important if participants were to benefit from home visits, instead of finding them a monitoring
gesture. The difference between cultural stereotyping/pigeonholing and cultural
sensitivity was identified as the former assumes that 'heard' cultural knowledge
applies to all while the latter takes the individual's cultural context seriously
(Ferns, 2005).

Participants valued the meeting spaces provided by statutory services and
community organisations. The connectedness fostered enabled them to keep
updated about information such as access to available services as well as joining in social activities that could provide a structure to their daily lives. Fear
of gossip emerged as a barrier to building connectedness, because of not being
able to reciprocate given persisting symptoms and the differences of cultural
practices within Chinese communities. Despite the importance of connectedness to participants, they experienced valued services being cut as contracting
funding and changing commissioning policies impacted on the capacity of
voluntary organisations to provide sustainable services. For participants who
encountered structural barriers to the expansion of their lives and relied on
community support, this contraction of services threatened to diminish their
connectedness.

This chapter also looked at ideological, institutional and structural levels and asked to what extent participants life chances had recovered and/or
increased to live the life they want to have. One positive factor was the increase
in positive freedom of carers and some overseas brides as the result of psychological work that helped them build their self-esteem and self-worth to realise
a life they valued (Zimmermann, 2006). Paid employment could be economically and psychologically empowering. However, the demands of gendered
caring and housework still confined the opportunities of some participants to
build a life outside domesticity. In other arenas, participants experienced various dimensions of exclusionary force (Ratcliffe, 2004). Exclusionary force
operates at a transnational level. Disadvantages relating to gender inequality
and mental health stigma experienced in the home country and barriers to
re-inclusion means that staying in the UK might be the only available or preferred option. In the case of asylum seekers, who had the lowest capabilities

set and lived at the margins of society, gaining a legal residence status opened up a recovery space.

The exclusionary forces experienced in the labour market and workplace was acute. The hegemony of normativity in ableism and sanism intersected with capitalism to disadvantage service users who already experienced racism. The narratives of Ken, Young and Lai-Ming illustrated how ableism operated. The driving force of capital accumulation in for-profit sectors discouraged the employment of people who experienced biographical disruption because of ill health and restricted the notion of acceptable work performance. The protection afforded by disability discrimination legislation had no effect in the experience of participants.

Feng's narrative demonstrated the operation of sanism. While he was able to do the physical work required of him in the workplace, he took self-limiting measures to prevent the 'slip' of his abnormal or 'mad' thoughts. Not only was the loss of capability due to exploitative working conditions difficult to recover from, the barriers in the labour market and workplace resulted in pro-longed unemployment for some participants led to further capabilities loss. The structural exclusionary force resulting from the ingrained ableism and sanism in the labour market meant that employment programmes aiming to increase the skills of disabled people had limited scope to effect changes in increasing their chances of employment. The limitations on participation in economic activities means that benefits were important for the survival of participants. However, the benefit system and the 'anti-scrounger' discourse contributed to participants' sense of vulnerability and reinforced the disciplining effects of being rendered incapable.

Compared with the social locations of the participants in pre-recovery as discussed in Chapter 3, the narratives of the participants and the structural barriers they encountered when trying to exercise their agency resulted in the emergence of new social locations. The negative aspects of the pathologisation process as well as sanism and ableism shown in this chapter intersected with the generative mechanisms arising from gender, class and ethnic inequalities. The new social locations, and the new capabilities sets they experienced and perceived impacted on the shaping of participants' worldviews along their recovery journey. The next chapter reveals how the participants made sense of their recovery, their notion of hope and its relationship to adaptive preferences.

6   Stubbornly strive to be human

Meanings of recovery, hope and
adaptive preferences

Introduction

The previous chapters have explored and analysed what participants recovered
from and the social conditions they recovered into. The participants' narratives showed how they had tried to get back to the helm and steer through the
obstacles and turbulence they encountered during this process. In this chapter I
will illuminate how the participants made sense of the direction in which their
lives were travelling. It builds on the discussion of the new social locations the
participants found themselves in, as well as how they reflected on their recovery journeys in terms of their evaluation of their present circumstances, future
chances and life plans. The life strategies they employed in maintaining and
asserting agency in the face of a sense of entrapment as well as pursuing a valued
way of life are analysed (Wong and Tsang, 2004; Welzel and Inglehart, 2010).
The concept of hope, a key component in the recovery approach (e.g. Deegan,
1996a; Russinova, 1999; Repper and Perkins, 2003), will be used in this chapter,
drawing on the participants' narratives and linking them to agency and adaptive
preference (Parse, 1999; Khader, 2012).

   Hope has been discussed as a psychological capability that stimulates recovery and personal change to counteract hopelessness and pessimism (Russinova,
1999). It has been understood in various ways, such as a capacity to aspire and
a sense of possibility (Ware *et al.*, 2008), a belief in self (Deegan, 1996a), or
closely related to the meaning and value of life (Landeen *et al.*, 2000). The
importance of hope or future orientation in facilitating the recovery journey is
about more than stressing the possibility of an optimistic recovery outcome – it
is central to humanity. Deegan (1996a) poetically linked hope with humanity and
argues this is where the recovery approach differs from the rehabilitative model.

> Many of us find this connotation of the word rehabilitation to be oppressive.
> We are not objects to be acted on. Rather we are fully human subjects who can
> act, and in acting can change our situation. We are not objects to be fixed. Such
> a connotation robs us of our own sense of autonomy and self-determination. It
> places responsibility in the wrong place. It perpetuates the myth that we are not
> and cannot be responsible for our own lives, decisions and choices.
>
> (Deegan, 1996a: 11)

In other words, hope and future orientation is important for service users to exercise agency in order to steer towards a life they want to pursue.

The discussion of hope in the recovery literature has addressed the necessity for mental health systems and professionals to nurture hope and aspiration so that service users can develop capabilities to realise their potential. Yet hope as a social construct can be experienced as capability diminishing and agency limiting, as it is shaped by oppressive ideologies and conditioned by social structures. Therefore, alongside participants' experiences of mental health services, evidence about how social conditions shaped the meaning of hope and how the notion of hope can be capability enhancing or limiting is considered (Onken *et al.*, 2002). Parse (1999) described how hope could be experienced:

> The meanings of hope described by participants are their structured realities arising in conforming-not-confirming cherished beliefs with speaking-being-silent and moving-being-still. Unique rhythmical patterns of relating as described by participants are paradoxical, incarnating being with and away from close others, while living all-at-once the opportunities and restrictions of pushing onward with the expanding horizons that unfold with new endeavors.
>
> (Parse, 1999: 288)

Participants' articulated hope related to their structured realities involves participants' subjective assessments of their social locations. Looking at the lived experience of hope opens up the exploration of the dynamic of the agency–desire adaptive preference social condition. This is where articulated hope, the presence or absence of life goals and having the will to hope leads to the flourishing or expansion of capabilities. How this relates to unequal and oppressive conditions is also important to explore (Khader, 2012). In this chapter, themes are generated from an analysis of participants' experiences of, and reactions to, sanism and ableism, formation of hope, adaptive preferences, strategies in steering life and aspiration to develop agency.

Sanism and the use of identities as life strategies

While sanism operated at a structural level in limiting participants' life chances in pursing a valued life, Chapter 5 showed how recurrent the notion of normalcy, i.e. a divisive line about what are normal behaviours, was in participants' narratives. The effect of sanism was experienced as an invalidation at the social-existential level (Pilgrim, 2008). Illness, disabled and service user identities were developed and employed as adaptive strategies, consciously or otherwise, as a defence against such invalidation during day-to-day encounters. These identities, in turn, shaped the development of participants' future orientation.

Invisibility and visibility: sanism, normalcy and experience of invalidation

Ignorance, prejudice and discrimination are barriers to participants trying to convert their social capital into capabilities (Thornicroft *et al.*, 2007). Danny and Lai-Ming experienced direct attacks. Danny thought that people discriminated against him as they only noticed him when he lost temper but did not notice that he was ill and depressed. Lai-Ming relied on children to tell him when he was not looking well, in his words 'behaving strangely'. However, at times he felt that he was just expressing his emotions while other people called it 'behaving strangely'. He used a disabled identity to resist such attacks instead of complying with discrimination.

> When people see you and realise . . . that you are not that normal. Abnormal. People say 'You are crazy'. I think to myself, 'I am not crazy'. I feel upset by it. When people say you behave strangely like this or that. But I think 'No, I am not'. I feel irritated by what they say. For example, when people laugh at you, of course I feel sad. I am crazy, but don't tell me that I am crazy. Like if people point out that you are crippled or you are deaf, it hurts. No one wants to have a disability.

While Wu-Wei and Carol did not experience direct attacks from acquaintances and strangers, they restricted their movements in order not to expose their vulnerability. Wu-Wei felt the weight of recovering from the aftermath of an episode during which she talked to neighbours about how she could save the world. Carol had experienced panic attacks and uncontrollable crying on buses. So on days that she felt she might have a crying spell, she would not go out in order to 'avoid embarrassment'. In this way Carol retained her pride.

Participants found maintaining social relationships difficult. Marcus and Carol used flexibility as a strategy to avoid exposing his symptoms and drawing attention to his ill health. When arranging to meet people they tried to keep the arrangements open. Yet, trying to use flexibility as a self-care strategy has its costs. As Marcus put it,

> This illness I think is complicated. Because you don't know when you are well and when you are not. You don't dare stressing yourself. So everything has to be flexible and skillful. But if you try to be flexible, you will still worry a lot by managing the schedule. So it feels like a vicious cycle.

The worries that accompany flexibility include having to establish an understanding with the person being met as well as negotiating an arrangement they will agree to. To Marcus, such worries could result in insomnia and headaches.

Invalidation does not only happen because of visible differences. While such differences made participants feel embarrassed enough not to socialise with people, the invisible dimensions of mental health difficulties also drove some participants to isolate themselves when their acquaintances casually dismissed their difficulties.

During the interview Feng stressed how different he felt he was from other people. It was as if he had to be clear and simultaneously defend himself about looking normal, in case I did not believe he was ill. He was not sure if he would ever become normal again.

> I want to recover mentally, but I don't know . . . I don't know how to recover. But I know this illness. I appear normal. But when I get home, I look different. My glance and my movement will be a bit . . . lunatic. I feel a bit blank. It's different. I feel different.

Hiding mental health problems can be painful. Rachel had opportunities to meet people who were not service users through art classes. However, she preferred to hang out with people with mental health difficulties as she thought it was 'easier'. Author: Easier in what way?

Rachel: To socialise because they've gone through similar things.
Author: What do you think you have in common with them? What are the similar things?
Rachel: I think the same experience of getting over schizophrenia. It helps socialising. But not with old friends because they don't understand it.
Author: Have you tried?
Rachel: Yes.
Author: What were their reactions?
Rachel: They thought I am ok. But I don't feel I am ok.
Author: They don't understand?
Rachel: Because sometimes I write things and my mind goes somewhere else. Sometimes I write strange stories. Like I say things that are not real, although in my mind it seems real.

It was not only friends that participants found did not understand them. Marcus told friends in mainland China about his mental health difficulties. However, they dismissed what he told them and said, as they laughed, 'if you have mental illness, we also have mental illness'. This reaction could reflect perceptions in mainland China that the overseas Chinese in the UK are living a better life, as Marcus thought they did not believe that he experienced difficulties. It also reflected the ignorance of his friends about the variety of ways mental ill health presents as well as their stereotypes of what a mental health patient looks like. Their dismissal and teasing had a silencing effect. Marcus did not mention his problems to his friends again.

Oa-Yeung was the one participant who did not mind sharing her thoughts. She was not worried about what other people thought or understood. Speaking her mind was important to her. Other participants tried to monitor themselves and be strategic in disclosing their diagnosis or sharing this part of their life with others.

However, this did not always work, as Ken explained. He did not usually mention his mental illness to friends. 'I don't mind people knowing it. But sometimes I don't know what to say, because they don't understand our situation. They think we are lazy and not bothered to work.'

However, Ken sometimes felt the need to tell people that he had a mental health problem overwhelming. Interestingly he called this need a symptom,

> I have found that since I have had mental illness, I want to talk to people about it. I want to tell people I have mental illness, so that people can be more sympathetic to me. My uncle took me to meet his friends. I suddenly told these people who I just met the first time that I had mental illness. It was out of the blue.

Usually cautious about keeping his mental illness from acquaintances, Ken found that he could not suppress his voice all the time. Calling this behaviour a symptom seemed to imply that it was impossible for him to suppress his need to be understood. This seemed to be an unconscious way of dealing with the invalidation he had experienced.

Ken: My uncle reacted quickly. He said someone who had mental illness would not say he had mental illness.

Author: How did you feel?

Ken: Of course I didn't buy it. I just wanted to tell them that I had mental illness. So that they . . . I don't mind how they thought of me. But they thought I was joking.

Author: How did you react next?

Ken: How I reacted next? Nothing special. I prefer to tell the truth. I prefer to tell the truth no matter if you accept it or not. I tell the truth and this is the truth. But they thought people with mental illness wouldn't tell others they have mental illness. Things like that.

Author: But you didn't explain the truth to them.

Ken: No.

All these ways of dealing with other people show how participants dealt with the social realm. They had restricted space to be themselves in. This restricted sense of space reflected a restriction of their capability to be at ease with themselves as service users and rebuild their lives after the shipwreck. Feeling unable to suppress telling others about oneself, without bothering with justifications, shows the strength of an individual's agency. It is like grass shoots growing out of a heavy concrete wall.

This restricted sense of being, experienced by participants in their daily lives, illustrated the effects of the exclusionary force of the ideology of normality in social interactions. It is in the process of learning to handle this weight that service users developed their future orientation on their recovery journeys, adapting their life goals in relation to the entrapment they experienced due to the restrictions of their existence. Participants' narratives showed the differing ways of using their ascribed identity of patienthood, disablement and being service users to adapt their lives.

Using illness, disabled and service user identities against invalidation

The ways participants used illness identity, disabled identity and service user identity as responses to the invalidation they experienced could be considered as an adaptation. It showed how they were striving for a space in which they could exist. Feng stressed repeatedly in his interview how he was not normal anymore.

> From what you see I look ok. I talk with you. It appears that I talk normally. But I really have problems. I really am ill. Today I talked to you, I told you everything I experienced. I am less severe than before. I didn't want to talk to people before. Although I may appear OK to you, I know very well that I have an illness.

Feng considered he was ill because his thinking was not 'normal enough'. He used an illness identity to communicate the invisible distress he experienced. He used the sick role to create a space for existence despite the invalidation he experienced socially (Gerhardt, 1979; Parsons, 1975; S.J. Williams, 2005). Taking on the sick role (as shown in Chapter 5) was his way of managing his symptoms. He was careful and took small steps to take on manageable challenges so as not to overstress himself and avoid a relapse. It was also a way to defend his benefit claiming against the anticipation of being called a benefit scrounger. With medicalisation being the characteristic feature of mental health promotion campaigns in the UK, Hong Kong and many other countries, Read *et al.* (2006) comment that adopting a sick role is a socially sanctioned way to live alongside sanism, an alternative to subverting it.

However, the sick role can be capability diminishing in the way it individualises a social problem as personal pathology, resulting in self-surveillance and self-accusation. As shown in Chapter 5, instead of thinking that his bullying and stigmatising working environment was the problem, Feng considered not being able to work in it was his problem. Similarly Ken had to deal with the effects on others of his adoption of a sick role. In talking about the next step in his recovery journey, Ken said he lacked the motivation to find work. He put it down to a psychological symptom he had – 'hesitation to find work' – which he tried to tackle with counselling. 'This is one of my symptoms. I mean I only talk the talk. Up till now I could not make it happen. I only have a vague idea of what kind of jobs I could find.'

Ken did go to the job centre to look for job openings, and he had been interviewed for an IT job, which he later realised required him to put money into training before being officially employed. Given this, what did he mean by lacking the motivation to find work? What held him back, he said, was having to go to the toilet frequently, which he suspected was a side effect of his medication. He was also reluctant to work in Chinese catering because it involved working long hours. He worried that his life would be boring with such work. To understand what he meant by boring and the unpleasant future it implied, it is important to put Ken's recovery journey in the context of his life history. He had started to change his career path as well as do things he took a genuine interest in before his breakdown. For example, he tried jobs with more human contact, such as teaching. He had taken a 'gap year' to attend creative writing classes, which he found meaningful. After his breakdown, Ken made a conscious decision not to hurry into employment. He had been relying for a living on his savings and earnings from the part-time work he did for friends. At the time of his interview, he thought it was 'about time' to get a job. However, he could not bring himself to apply for one.

Ken: I worry that I would feel bored after getting a job.
Author: What do you mean by 'bored'?
Ken: Now I go to my friend's house sometimes to have dinner with his family. Also every week I visit another friend – I call her grandma, she reads and comments on my creative writing. I think that if I do get a job, I would have to give up these activities. Life would be boring. These activities keep me alive. So if I go to work every day, going to work and then going home. It would be boring.

His 'lack of motivation' was in fact a very human resistance to the alienation he had experienced at work during his years in the IT sector.

Ken: A lot of my past work experience was very boring and rigid. When the company gave me some projects to lead, I might have some sense of achievement. But otherwise I felt bored.
Author: Did you like the nature of that work?
Ken: Actually I only worked for a livelihood. The working hours were long. Also it was very boring. Most of the time I worked on my own and I had to wait until colleagues went home to fix their computers. Also you know in an office there are lots of politics. But we don't have choice, do we? We have to pay the rent and fill our stomachs. So there was not much satisfaction so to speak. I just read novels as a past time to balance my life.

Ken's reference to a 'lack of motivation to look for jobs just for their instrumental values' as a symptom reflected the internal tug of war he was having about maintaining control over his working life so that it was meaningful and gave him satisfaction. Calling it a symptom could be read as a metaphorical way of understanding his situation. However, in Ken's case, it posed the question as to whether pathologising this human quest to engage in meaningful and creative work, by calling it a symptom, contributed to his capability development. Solutions to pathologisation, such as counseling or joining employability programmes, focused on 'fixing' individuals. However, the diversity of jobs that Ken referred to called for the expansion of opportunity structures at a societal level, i.e. a change in the socio-economic structure (Orton, 2011). Ken's valued doing and being, such as creative writing and his wish to run a tai-chi class in the park that people could freely join, may not be productive in economic terms but make a contribution to his flourishing as well as a potential contribution to the collective capabilities of his community.

Taking on a disabled identity was another way to live alongside sanism. Lai-Ming talked about how his doctor said his behavior was abnormal and how he had come to equate abnormality with illness and disability.

> Yes. It's a disability, isn't it? It's a disability. I admit it. Every illness is a disability. Doctor said that yelling at people means you are abnormal. He asked why I suddenly yelled at people. A normal people won't yell at people. People who yell at people are not normal. It's not normal behaviour.

In the face of the prejudice Lai-Ming experienced, as described above, he followed a script of medicalisation and pathologisation as defence. However, this strategy seemed to have another consequence, as his words indicated. He seemed to police the expression of his own emotions under what sanism validated and limited (Poole *et al.*, 2012).

Jerry took on a service user identity and thought that this identity had deepened over the years. This identity was not arisen from the invalidation he had experienced from acquaintances. It had come from the invalidation he had experienced from, in his words, the 'elements of control' in the mental health system.

Jerry: Actually I think psychiatry is complicated, there are many rules and medications. People who haven't experienced this can't really put themselves in the shoes of this community, the psychiatry community. A lot of doctors don't bother.
Author: They didn't listen to you carefully?
Jerry: They are bored about us. Having to listen to us all the time (laugh). Prescribe medications. Keep taking medication. Otherwise you will deteriorate.
Author: So it's different from what you want from them.
Jerry: Yes.

In talking about his future plans, Jerry revealed what he wanted and his recovery goal. In the long run he wanted to be able to move on and work. Yet the messages he got from professional stressed maintenance through medication rather than hope.

Jerry: I need to recover fully first before I consider that route (work).
Author: What do you mean 'recover fully'?
Jerry: Like I don't have to live in those hostels. That I can earn money. I don't have to take so many medications. Adjust . . . Don't have to take so many.

Author: Does it have any side effect, your medication?

Jerry: Taking medications makes you tired. Taking it for a long time makes you weak. Very tired. I usually take it at 8pm. To help me sleep.

Author: Has anyone, social worker or doctor, helped you achieving these aims?

Jerry: I don't know. I don't see them regularly. It's the hostel manager who sees me more frequently.

Author: Does he give you advice?

Jerry: No, no. Just tell me to take the medication.

His service user identity came with an awareness of power disparity in the mental health system. This led him to feel that he had to study mental health-related legislation to know about his rights and entitlements in order to protect himself in the mental health system and build his future.

The formation of hope and adaptive preferences

Participants did not only form and draw on illness, disabled and service user identities as strategies against invalidation and reassessing their future. Some also drew on other sources in shaping their hope and life plans. Religious faith and popular culture were mentioned as two such sources.

Religious faith as a source of hope

Hins and Raymond mentioned religious faith as their source of hope. As shown in Chapter 3, Raymond said his hope to go to university 'was dead'. Feeling frustrated by the loss of a hope that had given direction to his life, he went to church and found religion gave him something to believe in. 'It's better for me. If I have no hope there's no point in living in a way. If there is something to look forward to in the end, then it's worth fighting for.'

Hins, feeling certain that she would not relapse again, quoted Christian faith as her source of strength. Her understanding of Christian teaching gave her resilience because of the future it promised.

> In the past when I encountered things I would be lost. But after believing in God, I know I will go to a very good place in the future. In the Bible it talks about heaven. It doesn't only mean that you go to heaven after death. Living on the earth as if living in the heaven. When you have God in your heart, your life will be like in heaven. It's not something empty. You have hope. It really helps me solve a lot of things.

Apart from having a hope or vision of her future, the meaning of life had changed for her because of her belief in God. Before this she had wondered why she had been 'the unlucky one'. Now she viewed setbacks as tests in growing up and she felt able to accept them. Bible teachings, such as loving and forgiving your enemies, provided her with guidance about how to resolve the seeds of hatred sown in her because of being bullied at school. She felt that she could trust God because people could retaliate but God would never leave her. She felt that her relatives defined her in relation to the memory of her aggressive behaviour before she went to hospital when she was a child. She also felt that her mother could not let go of the past. Having been diagnosed with schizophrenia and admitted to a psychiatric hospital was a big thing for her mother who would remind Hins about it when recalling how her precious baby girl encountered a difficult life. 'But I really didn't like to hear about it. Because I believe in God now. I am a new person. I don't want to look back. But she always mentions it.'

For Hins, a new identity of being a dedicated Christian allowed her to put the past behind her. As discussed in Chapter 5, Hins was mentally well and was not on long-term medication. Yet, the discrimination she experienced from her kinship network seemed to have entrapped her by identifying her with her past history of mental ill health. Recovery, to her, was about personal transformation, asserting a new identity for herself and the people around her. Religious belief, apart from providing an anchor, provided her with the resources to narrate a new chapter in her life.

When hope can be capability diminishing: norms that construct disappointment

Like Hins, Tang-Yung also wanted to distance herself from her illness identity. She disliked the feeling of patienthood that she associated with a sense of victim-hood. 'I had to take an injection all the years. This makes me feel that I am ill, that I have been always ill. I felt unhappy about this.'

It seems that while Tang-Yung refused to identify with pathologisation, she embraced a dominant gendered ideology of the 'good life' fuelled by consumer-ist culture. She liked watching television programmes about fashion and glamour and explicitly related them to hope.

Author: How does it make you happy?
Tang-Yung: The fashion is pretty. The models are pretty on the catwalk. I like to watch it. I feel that there is some hope in life watching it.

Such hope, however, caught Tang-Yung in a vicious cycle of disappointment and hope. On the one hand, it seemed to give her something to aspire to, 'I want to wear those clothes on television. I want to fight for myself.'

On the other hand, the ideal set by this glamorous celebrity culture fed the idea of being 'not good enough'. She had ambivalent feelings towards this kind of hope. The more she hoped, the more upset she was about the weight gained due to her medication and unhealthy diet. She despised herself for being too fat to squeeze into the size zero clothes on television. Although she could not fit into the branded clothes she had brought for herself, she hung on to them.

Tang-Yung said she had not been into buying clothes in the past. The formation of her preference for pretty clothes and a glamorous lifestyle was illustrative of the 'evaluation anxiety' prevalent in unequal societies. This is a vulnerability that, Wilkinson and Pickett (2011) argue, is characteristic of a modern psychological condition that feeds into consumerism. Tang-Yung's evaluation anxiety intersected with gender, ethnicity, class and age inequalities. She felt that she was caught in a serial disappointment. She came to the UK to find that the man who she thought was her husband was already married. She left him and moved into her own home but a burglary took away all her possessions. Her new partner cheated on her like her ex-husband did. She said it was after the burglary that she started buying brand-named clothes she could not afford and she got into debt. Since then she found this spending habit hard to break. She compared herself with people around her, for example, migrants who came to the UK at the same time as she had and had built successful businesses and lived in big houses. Her mother in China told her not to compare herself with these people. But Tang-Yung felt that her family were the ones who compared her with other people, as they liked to talk about getting rich. Living in the UK, seeing people shopping and on television programmes, she wanted to be a celebrity and did not want a life without money or status. She called her obsession with pretty clothes her hope, but at the same time Tang-Yung said she knew that possessing lots of clothes did not give her the satisfaction she craved for. 'Sometimes I think I've got nothing in my life apart from the fat on my body.'

She shared this with her community nurse, who then told the doctor that she wanted to be a celebrity. 'That's how she talked about me,' said Tang-Yung, feeling that she was being laughed at. She was also given an injection that she was told would help her curb her spending. She did not think it had helped. Friends in the community centre had encouraged her to reduce the time she watched television. These individualistic responses failed to help her deal with her deep-seated feeling of social distance and evaluation anxiety.

Tang-Yung's aspiration to be a celebrity as a way out of her current life is one that is endlessly promoted in the UK and other parts of the world, including China. Reality shows give hope to ordinary people that they too can be a star. At the same time they reaffirm and reinforce the social distance between the successful achievers and the have-nots. Individual attempts to build resilience against this promotion of consumerism by the mass media face difficulties because of the economic power of global media conglomerates. As Evans points out (2002: 59), 'Centralization of power over the cultural flows that shape preferences is a more subtle form of "unfreedom" than those which Sen highlights, but no less powerful for being subtle'. In other words, the hope of becoming a celebrity, promoted by mass media as a way out of entrapment in life, limits an individual's capabilities and effective freedom. Development of collective capabilities is required to counter the hegemony of celebrity and consumerist culture for sustainable and achievable preferences to be pursued.

At an individual level, Tang-Yung's clearly articulated hope could be considered as an adaptive preference as it seemed to hinder, rather than foster her flourishing. This presented a challenge in empowering Tang-Yung to embrace a hope that was capabilities enhancing and contributive to well-being, while not negating the way Tang-Yung was hanging onto this hope and depriving her of 'what she had left' in her life (Khader, 2011).

Cautious strategies in steering life

Some participants were more cautious about speaking of hope than Hins and Tang-Yung. This caution did not mean that they were less determined to recover. Instead, it was a strategy directed at preserving resilience in living with distress, ill health and invalidation.

A measured hope and 'normal life': a balancing act in life planning

To Rachel, having a routine and taking care of herself to avoid a relapse were all part of what normal life meant to her. 'I just take medication . . . and try to do as much as I can with volunteering. Medication and volunteering help me get back into a routine. They help me with a normal life.'

Rachel also maintained this normal life by trying to avoid people who she perceived were not able to relate to her.

Rachel: Yes I stop being involved with high school friends. University college friends. I don't see them anymore. I don't actually do much artwork outside. Anywhere outside [the town]. I might write strange things. Draw strange things.

Author: You are worried?

Rachel: Yes a bit worried. That's why I need someone to read through things with me. I can read it but I may not be concentrating. I find it quite difficult.

Author: You are worried about what other people would think?

Rachel: Yes I think so. Yes.

Rachel seemed to be very careful in maintaining a normal life through restricting her social circle. At the same time she had tried to explore possibilities to pursue her desire to work in design, which was in line with her interests and talent in the arts, the subject she read at university. However, even if she felt able to move beyond her worry about other people, there were other barriers to working towards the realisation of this desire. She avoided travelling far. She did not think she could cope with travelling on a train by herself or taking a bus journey that required a transfer. She said that she would get anxious, as she could not cope with a long journey that required processing information such as timetables and reading routes. This seemed to relate to her bad memories of getting lost on trains during her breakdown. She would only travel in groups, such as on the outings organised by the outpatient clinic. On top of her fear of travelling was her concern about money. She said she would not travel to central London to visit the museums that she loved because the fares were high. Because she lived in a town where there were few art studios, these barriers to travelling meant that Rachel was not able to access the opportunities to study design by going to classes or working in studios in other towns or cities

Lai-Ming had begun a distance-learning course but gave it up. 'I didn't finish the course. I thought I'd better not give myself too much stress, it's not good to breakdown again. It's not a good time to break down. So I gave up the study.' The phrase 'it's not a good time to break down' summarised the balancing act that Rachel and Lai-Ming were involved in as they lived their lives. They moved between attempts to stretch their lives and avoid relapses. It is through this kind of balancing that adaptive preferences are formed and life goals are reviewed. The possibilities for Rachel to realise her desire were limited to helping, unpaid, in a local art class. Lai-Ming had reached retirement age and had not been able to work for some years. While he was clear that the jobs he might get would be one-off jobs paying an honorarium in the voluntary sector, he still went to the job centre regularly. He said it was like 'going to therapy' and tried to increase his employability by taking English language tests and honing his Chinese calligraphy skills to target jobs in the mainstream labour market and 'niche' Chinese communities. To balance disappointment and perseverance, Lai-Ming embraced Chinese proverbs such as 'there are no flowers that blossom forever' (*Hua wu bai ri hong*) to keep him going.

Between hope and daring not to hope

Carol found it difficult to deal with the pressures of housework while having to cope with her fluctuating symptoms (for details see Chapter 5). When I asked what recovery meant to her, she linked it to a 'cured' state in which she would be symptom-free and medication free. This resonates with the notion of 'recovery from illness', in contrast to 'recovery from impairment' and 'recovery from invalidation' (Pilgrim, 2008: 297). Yet, her doctor told her to be prepared to take medication for life.

> Recovery means I won't need to take medication. I don't need to have panics or anxiety. If I don't need to take tranquillisers or any other medication, this means I recover. But my doctor told me once 'you have to prepare that this illness will follow you the rest of your life. Till the day you die. You will still need to take medication'. I prepare for this to happen. But sometimes my son asks me, 'mommy, when can you stop taking medication? I really don't want you to die soon'. My heart sinks.

Her doctor had told her that the side effect of her long-term medication was the risk of early onset dementia. She was upset about this as she wished to attend her son's university graduation ceremony when he grew up. Carol's desired state of 'being' was to be symptom and medication free, but it was not an end in itself. I asked what she would like to do if one day she did recover as she defined it and did not have to take medication anymore.

A lot of things! First, I want to get a driving licence! Why? My husband does not let me do it, because he worries that when I have a relapse I may disappear. He worries that I would crash and die. I understand fully where his concern comes from. So if I really can recover, I will try to get a driving licence because I really look forward to driving my son around and showing him things. The joy of showing him the world. I also want to leave the UK. I really hate living in the UK. I really wish my son grows up soon so that I can retreat to Hong Kong.

These two wishes reflect Carol's aspiration to exercise her agency and that she considered her agency to be contingent on her well-being. The two things she wanted to do, i.e. literally be in the driving seat to drive her son around and move back to her home country, can be understood as desiring freedom of movement. While it seemed that Carol had a clear sense of what she wanted for recovery, she seemed to be bouncing between hope and not daring to hope.

I have waited for many years. I really look forward the day I recover. I am wretched. The torture. You know these medications have a lot of side effects. My body has changed. My husband really wanted me to be cured. But I told him to give up. I can't be cured. The doctor gave up on me too. He only gives me pills. He just told me to try different pills.

Daring not to hope reflected her doctor's pessimistic attitude and became a coping strategy to avoid further disappointment in life, through hardening her heart (Deegan, 1996b). Speaking of her two wishes, Carol said,

But I dare not to hope such a perfect . . . or such a concrete plan . . . because even you just try to come up with a weekly plan, you may have a week of relapse. You won't know. So I really dare not to hope. And I also never thought of how real recovery would be.

To gauge the expectation of recovery, she used the notion of good relapses to make sense of the progress of the recovery. She would have a bad day of relapse and then could not recall what had happened during that day. Having relapses like this posed a psychological threat to her,

I would ask my husband, 'did I have a 'good relapse' yesterday? Did I shout at you two?' I was scared. It's a psychological threat to me. He would say, 'no problem! This time you handled it very well'.

The notion of a good relapse is used by Carol to retain a positive attitude to a recovery journey that can be fluctuating and grueling.

Compared to 6 years ago, I am still ill. But I am getting better, bit by bit. Every year, my birthday wish is to tell myself that I will recover. But I am getting tired now. A long-term battle. I really feel tired. Because you only have one brain but your brain can be divided into many parts to function. Like 70 per cent of your brain is having a relapse, fighting with the brain. With the remaining 30 per cent what do you have to do. What to do with this 30 per cent? I have to care for my son, the housework, my husband . . . I have no choice. Now I begin to learn to let go. For example, I used to argue with my husband. When I am angry now, I would tell myself, 'Please leave the fire for the other part of the brain, for the battle (against the relapse). Don't use the energy to fight with your husband. Otherwise I would have to take medications that wear me down. It's me who suffers eventually'. This is what I have learnt. I don't want to waste energy on trivial things. I am really tired.

Hence rationing her energy is another coping strategy Carol employed to deal with her daily household and caring work and internal turmoil.

As long as I have a path to walk along, I just walk. This is how I feel now. You can say I am pessimistic. I can tell myself 'Today is quite good! I didn't have a relapse! I earn a day'. This is how I think.

Aspiring to agency development and emancipation

Some participants did not talk about an explicit recovery goal or life goal. However, their narratives would often reveal a worldview that showed their desires, hidden aspirations in life, and glimpses of their desire for emancipation (Welzel and Inglehart, 2010). Young and Feng's aspirations for agency development could be understood in relation to the life stage they were at.

Transition into adulthood

Young's recovery journey had delivered downward social recovery as he said, 'I think my self-confidence is not up to me'.

He accepted that his persisting symptoms had to be managed through medication and had learnt how to cope when symptoms arose. So far his clinical recovery had been stable. However, he felt a great sense of loss and disempowerment from a journey begun at university, followed by negative work experiences and then being unemployed. Placing his recovery journey in the context of his life history showed that the increasingly lack of self-confidence he felt could be understood as a failed attempt to develop his sense of agency as a young adult.

Young: In the past I could make decisions. But now when working, I try to make decisions but it doesn't work . . . I had self-confidence in the past. I didn't think I would ever be ill. I had a lot of confidence before. When I started to get ill, the confidence disappeared.

Author: Over the years do you think your self-confidence come back, or further diminished?

Young: I think my self-confidence is not up to me . . . It's like I have to let other people make decision for me. May be they don't believe in me. Not many people accept this illness.

Author: Who do you refer to?

Young: They usually make decisions for me. Either 'go get a job' or 'go to study', telling me to take medication or not.

Author: *How does that make you feel?*

Young: Usually I have to listen to their advice. If I don't listen to them, it will hurt them.

The 'they' that Young referred to were his family. His issue of loss of confidence, which occurred at the beginning of his recovery journey and was not recovered over the years, had to be understood in the context of biographical time. His first breakdown happened as he was moving from late adolescence to adulthood (Shanahan, 2000). The way he described his confidence issues, not as a loss but as a thing that docs not bclong to him, revealed a deep sense of diminished agency. Falling mentally ill involves a deprivation of agency resulting in an inability to exercise mind and body to achieve desired 'doings'. For Young his unfinished undergraduate studies, the barriers he encountered at work and the pressures from his family added to the diminishment of his agency in shaping his biography. He said his confidence had increased 'a little bit' during the time he was going to a peer group at the Chinese community centre where he had learnt from others who were in the same situation. This suggested that learning about ways and strategies to aid recovery increased his feelings of being in control of his life.

Young felt that the pressures he had to deal with from his family were greater than the pressures he had experienced at work.

> Because close family members can hurt you. If you are hurt at work, you can understand it's just a job. But it is family, the relationship is deep . . . Maybe they are tired too. They may think I will never recover.

The barriers Young encountered in job seeking took a toll on his relationship with his family. He was aware of his parents' disappointments about his unsuccessful application for benefits. He thought his family did not understand him enough. Although his mother went to counselling at the Chinese centre with him, he said all she talked about was job seeking and benefits, which made him feel that she was talking about their private business.

Young: If I put the family pressure aside, I don't know what I am doing. Because every time it's my family suggests me to do things. I usually listen to them.

Author: Maybe it's about finding out what you really want?

Young: Yes. That's exactly what I lost.

Author: Maybe you can't find it in family?

Young: I have to find myself.

Young's reference to 'not knowing what he is doing' reflects a sense of losing his orientation in life. Diminished agency resulted in a loss in his bearings in relation to where he wanted his life to go. While he did not state any concrete hope about his recovery, his narrative suggested that he wanted to regain a sense of agency.

Not a life in a void: wanting to see the world

Feng did not have a concrete hope about his future either. The impression he conveyed was that he chose not to think too much about the future or how he envisioned his recovery. Instead he focused in the interview on the importance of maintaining his day-to-day mental well-being. Feng's breakdown happened when he was a young adult and his sense of the direction of his recovery can be understood in the context of his biography. He had sought better life chances when he risked entering the UK as an undocumented migrant. This better life was not just about economic improvement. He talked about how society is a university where one could see and learn a lot of things. Having been a young fisherman in a small fishing village in China, he felt that his years in the UK had broadened his horizons. He wanted to 'see the world' and carry on venturing in life.

> I learnt that the world is very big. There are a lot of things I haven't learnt. Because I had been staying in my own space . . . Firstly I can't speak English. Living in the UK without being able to speak the language . . . I do not think of going out to see this and that . . . But with the Chinese . . . those people at work . . . their mindsets are different. They just focus on work. They have their mindset. I have my own thinking.

Feng seemed to want to stop working in Chinese catering because the long working hours meant there was no time left for a personal life. However, his lack of language capability meant that this was difficult.

Feng: With this illness, if I carry on like this, I feel that life is meaningless. Although you have this psychological illness, you still have to accept this environment (living in the UK).
Author: What is a meaningful life to you?
Feng: I have not figured it out yet. For now I wish I to improve myself, I mean my psychological illness. It's how I think for now. If I have to live like this forever, my life will be a void.

Life with meaning was important for Feng, even though the content of the meaning was, as yet, unknown and he did not have a special goal to aim for. His aspiration seemed to have developed as a reaction to his alienating work conditions and his restricted social networks at this stage of his recovery journey. These intersected with his lower class background and marginalised positionalities within and outside Chinese communities in the UK. Not wanting to live a life in a void fuelled his perseverance to propel his recovery and life journey forward.

Conclusions

A recovery journey is an ongoing process. Its direction is a result of the structural forces an individual lives in and against, the resources they have and their aspirations in steering their life. This chapter focused on the participants' recovery journeys at the time of their interviews. The variations in the ways they asserted and exercised their agency in the face of structural constraints were illustrated. The invalidation that some participants experienced as a result of sanism and their feelings of entrapment at interactional and structural levels was detailed. Participants defended themselves against invalidation by adaptively taking up illness, disabled or service user identities. The use of these identities in turn shaped the way participants developed understandings of their predicaments, projected their future chances and orientated themselves in life.

In addition, the varieties of articulated hope and life plans reflected how social class, gender, ethnicity and ageism intersected in shaping the different ways cultural resources were used in envisioning lives. For example, the alienation Feng experienced working in restrictive and exploitative conditions fed his desire to explore the world one day. Social class played a part in reinforcing the social distance that Tang-Yung felt. Her attachment to fashion as a way to keep up appearances and her concerns with her weight were clearly gendered. Carol's desire to increase her freedom of movement, if a day came when her symptoms did not keep her at home, was linked to her mothering role. Hins and Lai-Ming illustrated different ways that belonging was experienced. While Hins wanted distance from the stigma she experienced from her kinship network in her home country, Lai-Ming embraced the cultural tradition of Chinese calligraphy to increase his chance of casual employment in Chinese communities in the UK and used Chinese idioms as a way to encourage himself in the face of setbacks and disappointments in life.

The analysis of the lived experience of hope in this chapter suggested that it was the agential aspect of hope that contributed to participants' capabilities development and enabled them to steer their lives with perseverance. The social conditions that enabled agency were conditions that provided a sense of the real possibilities for development and growth (Ware *et al.*, 2007). Sources that developed this sense of possibility were derived from possibilities sanctioned by the social structure. These were mediated by subjective life meanings and this explains how religious faith worked in facilitating recovery.

The findings presented in this chapter suggest further understanding of hope as a social construct in relation to social structure. The hope service users strongly embraced might not necessarily be capability enhancing enough for them to flourish. Tang-Yung's association of hope with the dominant ideology of success in popular culture reinforced a sense of impossibilities, keeping her in a cycle of disappointment. This suggests a need to be critical and collectively challenge the neo-liberal culture outside the mental health system – a culture that creates the mass failure of the weak while promoting the survival of the fittest through television competitions and reality shows.

On the contrary, when service users were cautious about articulating hope in terms of a concrete plan, they could be adopting 'strategies of existence' to actively negotiate their relationship to the world (Corin and Lauzon, 1994). Being cautious could be a way to slowly (re)develop their capabilities. As shown above, despite their seeming lack of a spirit of hope, these participants would reveal their inner aspirations when they were invited to reflect upon their wider life history. Thus their reservations about hope could be understood as an adaptive preference to avoid (repeated) setbacks and disappointment in the face of structural barriers in pursuing their life goals – an attempt to maintain control of their recovery journeys.

A final point could be made about the experience of hope. Comparing the debilitating hope that Tang-Yung articulated with the cautious gauging of hope by Carol and the preference of focus on day-to-day living that Feng adopted reveals a tension around hope. Such tension raises the question of whether the future-oriented mindset associated with hope could become a barrier for developing capabilities. Thích Nhất Hạnh, a Buddhist Zen master, suggests that while hope is important in helping us bear the hardships we experience, the emphasis Western civilisation places on hope can be an obstacle.

> Hope is for the future. It cannot help us discover joy, peace, or enlighten-ment in the present moment . . . I do not mean that you should not have hope, but that hope is not enough. Hope can create an obstacle for you, and if you dwell in the energy of hope, you will not bring yourself back entirely into the present moment. If you re-channel those energies into being aware of what is going on in the present moment, you will be able to make a breakthrough and discover joy and peace right in the present moment, inside of yourself and all around you.
>
> (Thích, 2010: 41)

This points to the possibility of developing alternative ways of nurturing agency and desires to foster the personal growth needed for a flourishing life.

7　Social conditions for recovery
Towards a social justice agenda

Introduction

This book began with a critique of the way the recovery approach was mainstreamed into mental health policy and services in the UK in the context of neo-liberal state policies. It highlighted how the resulting dominant discourse of recovery is individualistic, uses a narrow definition of recovery and fails to tackle the structural inequalities that contribute to distress and mental ill health in the first place and that can also hinder the recovery process. The aim of this study was to identify 'what people recover from' and turn it into an empirical inquiry that explored the interplay of structure and agency in enabling or constraining Chinese mental health service users to pursue and live a meaningful and valued life. This was achieved through proposing a framework based on the Capabilities Approach and Intersectionality Analysis, to analyse the data gathered through a case study of the recovery journeys of 22 Chinese people living in UK who had received a psychiatric diagnosis.

The common culturalist approach that perpetuates essentialism, homogenises diversity among members of minority ethnic communities or assumes the kind of life choices that are preferred, is unhelpful, even harmful, in understanding the variations of experience and the diverse needs of Chinese people in the UK. Thus I have demonstrated how to use the Capabilities Approach combined with Intersectionality Analysis to explore recovery and diversity. My argument is that it is necessary to understand the intersecting structural forces such as class, gender and ethnicity, without presuming that they wholly predetermine the destinations of service users' recovery journeys.

Three research questions guided this study. First, what are the Chinese mental health service users in this study recovering from and what do they recover into? This entailed looking at what contributed to their distress and mental ill health in the first place and what were the capabilities and life chances they strive to recover in order to rebuild a life along their recovery journeys. Second, what hinders and facilitates the recovery process, and in particular how do class, gender, ethnicity and other structural influences intersect to shape outcomes? In other words, how do such structural inequalities shape the direction of recovery journeys, by enabling or constraining service users' capability (re)developments?

Finally, what are service users' own assessments of their recovery journeys so far, in terms of the extent to which they consider themselves recovered and their hopes for the future? This last question focused on how service users made sense of their recovery journeys and whether their life goals were compromised and became 'adaptive' preferences because of the setbacks they have encountered in the past and the obstacles they anticipated in the future.

The remainder of this chapter is in four sections. The first section summarises the steps taken in Chapter 2 to formulate an alternative theoretical framework to address the three research questions. The second section argues that the rich data generated by this study reveal the complex and diverse way structural inequalities shape the social conditions in which Chinese service users in the UK recover and the different strategies they use to strive to move from patienthood to personhood. In the third section, the implications of this study for policy and practice are detailed. Finally, the chapter ends with a call to put social justice and tackling of social inequalities at the core of recovery agenda.

Exploring recovery, mental health and inequality with the Capabilities Approach and Intersectionality Analysis

Chapters 1 and 2 detailed how I built on concepts of agency developed from the recovery movement and used the Capabilities Approach and Intersectionality Analysis to form the theoretical framework for the study. To pave the way to answering the first research question 'From what to where?' with reference to what service user advocates propose in the recovery movement (Deegan, 1988; Ridgway, 2001), I asserted recovery as a non-linear continuing journey with a sense of movement from patienthood to personhood. The notion of a recovery journey was further elaborated borrowing metaphors used in the Tidal Model (Barker and Buchanan-Barker, 2005). The role of agency was discussed as critical to understanding why the directions taken in recovery journeys vary for each individual, and how service users strive to take control in steering the course they take, which is subject to currents from the oceans of experience.

The way currents from the oceans of experience, or social forces, impact on the shape of recovery journeys was demarcated into four phases, which were reflected in the organisation of Chapters 3, 4, 5 and 6. Chapter 3 looked at how social forces can contribute to distress and mental ill health resulting in a diminishment of capabilities to achieve daily functioning and life goals. Chapter 4 considered how the process of becoming a psychiatric patient can enhance or hinder the (re)development of capabilities relating to mental health. Chapter 5 detailed how social forces can facilitate or restrict the capability (re)development in rebuilding a life that the respondents in the study value along the recovery journey. Chapter 6 addressed how the Chinese mental health service users anticipate their future life directions.

In considering the second research question the choice and adaptation of theoretical frameworks was grounded in a critical realist exploration, which foregrounds analysis of material reality as well as culture. Distress and ill health were acknowledged as real while the way 'psychiatric disorder' is socially and historically constructed was critiqued (Pilgrim, 2015). Critical realism might share with postmodernist or 'strong' constructivism critiques of the dominance of the iatrogenic bio-medical model for its legitimacy and usefulness in understanding problems arising from the medicalisation of conditions such as sadness, hearing voices, anxiety, paranoia and incorrigibility. However, it differs from postmodernist or 'strong' constructivism by emphasising these conditions or 'symptoms' as real. This means that instead of deconstructing the 'medical' with the 'social', critical realism would explore the generative mechanisms that gave rise to these conditions or 'symptoms'. The complex interactions between social, psychological and biological factors would be explicated. Adverse life events and experiences, especially those experienced during childhood, render individuals more vulnerable to stressors. Thus, in this book, the analysis of 'what to recover from' started from exploring the context of the participants' life challenges, which then gave rise to their distress and ill health. Through this, the possible structural causation of the differences among the Chinese communities could also be brought to light. After establishing the critical realist framework, I moved on to explicate the use of the Capabilities Approach and Intersectionality Analysis in this study. I conceptualised the recovery journey from patienthood to personhood as a capability development. Using the Capabilities Approach in which capabilities were understood as 'substantive freedoms', comprising process and opportunities dimensions that allow freedom to act and decide and actual opportunities available for the valued doings and beings (Sen, 1999; Nussbaum, 2000; Hopper, 2007). The Capabilities Approach can accommodate diversity as it is not concerned with what a person eventually chooses to be or do, but whether a person has the capabilities to achieve it. Mental well-being is a valued state of 'being', it is also a capability with which a person can achieve other things. Thus the first research question was further explicated in terms of what capabilities were lost or deprived and what capabilities were (re)developed along the recovery journey.

The interplay between structure and agency was then explored through the life chances available to an individual. Thus I examined whether the agency of the individual is respected and there is scope for them to exercise it, and whether there are exercisable opportunities for them to achieve valued 'doings' and 'beings'. The role of conversion factors in the Capabilities Approach was also emphasised, for example, through examination of policies, welfare systems and legislation, all of which are barriers or facilitators for an individual to convert capabilities into 'doings' and 'beings'. The notion of adaptive preference was applied to the third research question in understanding how an individual can restrict or diminish their preferred life goals according to the barriers experienced and their perceived exercisable opportunities.

While the Capabilities Approach provides answers to what capabilities one needs to recover or develop, Intersectionality Analysis pushes the investigation towards asking why and how. How, for example, do class, gender, ethnicity, ageism, sanism and ableism, contribute to capabilities deprivation or constrain capabilities development? To tease out the complexity and variations of the interplay of structure and agency, the social location of Chinese mental health service users in the UK was explored from the outset. Social location was understood as 'translocational positionality' (Anthias, 2001, 2006). This emphasises the social position one locates in terms of social hierarchical intersecting structures, such as class, gender and ethnicity, embedded within and across geographical and national boundaries. It also refers to social positioning, i.e. the fluid ways one relates to cultural and social practices and identities. In terms of this study, it aimed to explore the fluid ways Chinese people relate to Chinese traditions and ethnicised ideologies.

The synthesis of the Capabilities Approach and Intersectionality Analysis led to the design of the methodology with life history as the primary data collection method. I used what I called 'translocational life history' to connect micro individual biography with macro social history and structure. Data collected with a translocational lens is capable of providing insight into the impact of the different inequalities in the national and transnational context of a person's biography.

Key findings: the capabilities loss and development of Chinese service users in the UK

Chapters 3, 4, 5 and 6 revealed that the life histories of the Chinese mental health service users in the UK participated in this study shared *a common humanity* despite variation in the directions of their recovery journeys. Their journeys showed how they strove, sometimes cautiously, to retain and exercise agency to move from patienthood to personhood. These journeys were shaped by social inequalities, demonstrating that targeting social inequalities is an inseparable part of facilitating and nurturing meaningful recovery. The invalidation experienced in the form of suppressed agency were common reasons for the extreme distress, bodily discomfort and inability to perform daily functions, which resulted in pathways to voluntary and involuntary mental health care. Capabilities deprivation generated by structural inequalities in the form of powerlessness, feelings of injustice and material deprivation were found to contribute to the mental health deterioration of participants.

Two key overarching themes emerged from the findings. First, *the participants' recovery journeys were shaped by capability deprivations resulting from the social conditions that contributed to their distress and mental ill health in the first place.* Therefore, to understand the social conditions that facilitate or constrain capabilities (re)development along the recovery journey (as shown in Chapters 3, 4 and 5), it is necessary to refer to, and tackle, the deleterious social conditions discussed in Chapter 3. Second, *along their pathway to care and in the process of rebuilding a life, participants encountered new capabilities deprivations.* They could be positioned in new social locations because, for example, of their entry into life course turning points or their entrapment in the discourse of abnormality and ableism. The new social locations they occupied resulted in new or added capability deprivations that they then had to recover from. While some Chinese service users in this study were able to develop the capability to deal with the predicaments that had contributed to their ill health, the social conditions they recovered in meant that there were often new challenges and capability deprivations that they then had to recover from. Accumulative capability deprivation could result in their opportunity gradient of life chances becoming steeper, which made the recovery project harder. A closer look at the interplay of structural inequalities and agency at different phases of the recovery journey was then taken.

When things started to fall apart: social conditions and capabilities loss

The social conditions leading to mental health deterioration that can be traced to structural ethnic inequalities at *national* and *transnational* levels were detailed in Chapter 3. For first-generation migrants, coming to the UK was anticipated to be an opportunity for capability development. However, for the migrants in this study, it was their deprived capabilities that resulted in limited coping resources and reduced chances to exercise agency. Language and citizenship were the two capabilities that were central to mental well-being. While the lack of the former was an impediment to the exercise of agency and access to available services and resources, the lack of the latter excluded undocumented migrants from the means of survival as they were exploited in exchange for shelter in 'hidden corners of society', mostly the Chinese catering business.

Mental health deterioration could be rapid for the second-generation Chinese service users in this study. While they did not have language or citizenship problems, their deprived capabilities could be socially transmitted from their first generation migrant parents. A family's lack of material resources meant economic hardship for the second generation. While the ethnicised and disaporic discourse of the Chinese 'valuing school', discussed by Archer and Francis (2006), is social and cultural capital that encourages the second generation to aim high in education, it can also be a source of considerable stress. Intergenerational conflict could occur if members of the second generation had different aspirations from their parents who wanted them to move up and away from their lower-class backgrounds. Psychological issues could arise from such intergenerational conflict and weakened family bonds. Thus relationships with parents and finding a life of their own were recurrent themes of 'recovery from' among these participants. In addition, this group's experiences highlighted the continuing effects of deprivation of mental health capability in young adulthood, a time crucial for capability development. Mental health crises while at university that resulted in dropping out meant that life chances in the job market were highly compromised. Lack of qualifications resulted in difficulty in finding skilled jobs, as evidenced in Chapter 5.

Gender intersected with ethnicity and class relations in shaping the social locations participants were positioned in. The deprived capabilities of migrants could be further traced to their gendered life course pathways. The themes of recovery were gendered. Gender ideology and gender structure shape participants' life chances and what they valued in life. Lower-class women who had migrated to the UK to marry often found themselves trapped in an isolated domestic sphere and experienced low self-esteem. While ethnicised gender ideology was used to justify their subordination to husband and family by older relatives, and sometimes by themselves, they also expressed aspirations to live a life for themselves. Thus this ideology, which they had adapted to and constrained their capabilities development, became what they had to recover from. The gendered pathway was also manifested in the impact of childbirth on women's mental health. The findings showed the limited social capital these women had within and outside Chinese communities that they could draw upon to cope with the demanding care of newborns and recovery from childbirth.

Male migrants' themes of recovery were dominated with the ways that work and the labour market adversely affected their mental health. In the UK they found themselves faced with a segregated labour market along ethnic and class lines. Even for those who could speak English, ethnic markers such as accent could be barriers to breaking into the mainstream labour market. Faced with the limited choice of working in the Chinese catering business, many talked about how their harsh working conditions contributed to their mental distress and ill health. Their low bargaining power at the workplace, i.e. limited agency, meant they had to cope with the work stress on their own, and the only way to deal with a mental crisis was to leave their job. The participants in these situations found capabilities related to work particularly difficult to recover from, as detailed in Chapter 5.

Becoming a psychiatric patient

Going through the psychiatric system could be capability enhancing as well as diminishing. Service users' pathways to health care and the process of medicalisation were scrutinised in Chapter 4, with a focus on what helps and what hinders in the recovery process. The use of Western and Chinese traditional medical models, in and outside UK and transnational health care systems, enabled some participants to get treatments that worked for them. Being able to be treated in their native language environment was felt by some to be a relief. It was important too, that participants felt their doctors from the statutory services were open-minded about different medical models and systems and were willing to facilitate their care in another country. Reassurance about their continued access to the public services if they sought help from the private sector was valued. The use by some participants of traditional Chinese treatments in the UK depended on whether they had the resources to pay for them. Making use of the transnational health care system depended on an individual's social capital in their home country, whether they could afford to travel, and whether they could be exempted for a while from their responsibilities in the UK.

Moving on from this discussion of the use of health care in general, the data analysis focused on the process of pathologisation and medicalisation of mental distress. Lack of English language capability emerged as the biggest hurdle for some migrants. The best interpretation services could deliver line-to-line interpretation, with an awareness of differences within the Chinese community and an ability to stay calm in distraught situations. Knowing the service users they were interpreting for was also identified as important by participants. However, even with good interpreters, participants felt that expressing their distress themselves was important in building a good working relationship with doctors. It seemed that talking to a doctor through a third person compromised participants' ability to assertively raise their concerns. Most importantly, seeking help for mental distress through interpreters appeared to hinder the process of making sense of a crisis, a process that was experienced as crucial to recovery.

Service users' experiences of the various elements of psychiatry, namely, diagnosis, medication, talking therapies and hospitalisation, were explored in the context of psychiatric power. The exercise of psychiatric power reflected in the imbalance of power between clinicians and service users with the former taking an authoritative and paternalistic role, as well as using their legal powers of involuntary admission, resulted in a denial of service user agency. This discouraged participants' proactive understanding and management of their condition. Such psychiatric power was deeply felt, especially by long-term service users, who became cautious in building a relationship with professionals and increasingly aware of their need to retain control of their lives.

The first element of psychiatry discussed was psychiatric diagnosis. The sick role sanctioned by a diagnosis was experienced by some participants as a way of getting a legitimate explanation of their distress and decreased daily functioning at the beginning of the medicalisation process. Knowing their diagnosis could also help participants educate themselves about their ill health using resources like the Internet. However, further along the recovery journey, sanism started to have a pronounced influence. This was experienced either in the form of outright discrimination, especially for those with highly stigmatised labels such as schizophrenia, or in being trapped in an abnormality discourse.

In terms of treatment and intervention, medication was usually the first and often the only treatment option offered to participants. All types of treatment, for example, medication or talking therapies, were considered as crucial to recovery by some and deemed useless by others. The side effects of medication became what some participants found they had to recover from. Patienthood experienced by users on long-term medication was a condition they said they wanted to recover from. The dismissal of service users' enquiries about medication, as well as past experiences of medication were identified by participants as hindering their effective use of medication. The use of medication was facilitated by those clinician who used a 'shared decision-making' approach in prescribing medication (Deegan and Drake, 2006). Clinicians who helped participants understand their prescribed medication especially by using a common language were valued.

In terms of talking therapy, users rejecting it were those who did not like to discuss their ill health with others and those who thought that the therapist would not understand their particular concerns. Therapy was welcomed by many women who as overseas brides had suffered from isolation and low self-esteem as a result of their entrapment in the domestic sphere and their burden of caring. The skills of the therapist were considered important while the costs of therapy, and the shortage of therapists speaking Chinese language and dialect were factors hindering their use.

Key factors that impacted on whether hospitalisation (voluntary or involuntary) was experienced by participants as contributing to recovery included the language environment of the hospital and whether participants got along with other service users. Staying in an unfamiliar institution uprooted participants from their living environments and this was experienced as being far from therapeutic. The subsuming of different cultural behavior and values under the process of micro-monitoring, using the lens of 'ab/normality' in hospitals was experienced as disabling.

It proved to be difficult to assert agency in a hospital setting. The denial of agency that was involved in compulsory admissions resulted in grievances, which could lead subsequently to the active avoidance of services. Denial of agency emerged as a factor that service users need to recover from. Only one participant considered his involuntary hospital admission useful. Prior to hospitalisation this participant suffered acute deprivation and denial of access to services because of his undocumented migrant status. Compulsory hospitalisation was considered useful by him because he had no other available option.

One important capability that was sidelined in bio-medical dominated psychiatry was the capability to make sense of the distress and ill health participants experienced. When the meaning-making process was considered important for recovery, they looked for an answer to the question 'why me?' and found that the sick role discourse could not provide a satisfactory answer. The co-existence of other explanatory models alongside medicalised understandings, as well as the rejection of medicalised understandings by some participants, pointed to the potential use of narrative therapy in the recovery process (Roberts, 2000).

Life after shipwreck: social conditions that facilitate or hinder recovery when rebuilding a life in the community

Participants used different kinds of statutory and voluntary services in rebuilding their lives. While home visits from the statutory services provided support to some participants after their hospital discharge, others felt that the workers who visited them were more interested in 'risk monitoring' (i.e. checking that they were not causing trouble to other people), rather than helping them (i.e. understanding and working with their needs). When being referred to community services, some bilingual participants felt disempowered as the workers would assume they prefer Chinese-speaking services instead of presenting them with options. They might want to distance themselves from certain Chinese cultural practices that they did not want to relate to. Assuming what bilingual Chinese service users need and prefer reflected a neglect of the agency of service users and failure to understand the changing nature of cultural practices and the fluid relationships service users have with cultural practices. One participant lived in a hostel where racism from other residents was rife. Although he aspired to an independent life, the pace of moving towards it was out of his control, as his social worker barely met up with him or discussed plans toward his independence. His social worker did not ask about his recovery goal.

Community meeting places in statutory and voluntary organisations for service users as well as members of the wider community were important spaces for recovery. Participants found that they could socialise with each other service users, participate in social activities and gradually rebuild their daily functioning at their own pace. Community centres and voluntary organisations were also important places for participants to obtain information about services, rights and entitlements. While such meeting places played an important role in empowerment and building the important capabilities of connectedness, participants were aware of the contraction of statutory services and how reductions in funding were negatively impacted on the sustainability of these valued places.

In addition to the availability of meeting spaces, there were other contributive factors in nurturing connectedness. Fluctuating symptoms could interfere with participants' ability to reciprocate in relationships. Some participants felt shy about using their social capital when they needed help, thinking of themselves as not being able to give anything back to friends in return. Reciprocity required an understanding of the variations in the codes of cultural practices that are to be found under the umbrella term of 'Chinese traditions'. Connectedness also requires being able to venture out into other social circles. Meeting places were a springboard for this, but connectedness also requires service users to have opportunities in other areas of life.

The transnational connections of migrants might suggest that they have the option of an alternative place to live 'back home'. However, such assumptions romanticise 'home' and ignore the inequalities that migrants face there. Inequalities that led them to migrate in the first place are what they might well encounter on their return. Because of this the possibility of capability development of migrants in the UK was an important issue. This was particularly relevant for the participants who were overseas brides, for whom an important recovery theme in their narratives was their development of self-worth. Overseas brides who equipped themselves with coping skills, for example, through talking therapies, and economic empowerment, were able to negotiate around their caring responsibilities and increase their status and position at home. However, the gendered division of work and their heavy household workloads were hindering structural factors that proved difficult for individuals to overcome, especially when they were struggling with persistent symptoms.

Employment was another important arena for capability development. Yet it also contributed to distress and could be an obstacle that hindered recovery. In a situation where one participant was able to keep their job after an acute crisis, the employer took a positive initiative; he kept in touch with the participant and did not rush her return to work. However, such good practice is difficult to find in the for-profit labour market, especially in Chinese catering businesses. While participants hoped for openness and diversity in the labour market, the reality they encountered was segregation. Being a member of an ethnic minority, in middle age and having a mental health history were all found to be significant disadvantages.

Sanism and ableism intersected with the logic of capital accumulation and reduced participants' chances of employment when competing in the ethnicised labour market. Participants who could speak English avoided the Chinese catering jobs that had made them ill in the first place. Participants who had had to drop out of studying because of ill health and lacked qualifications could only find low-skilled jobs with poor occupational safety and health. This resulted in a worsening of their mental health. 'Reasonable adjustments' sanctioned by anti-discrimination legislation did not happen for them. Users felt alone in negotiating in their workplaces and did not know whether a trade union could help when they felt they were being unfairly treated. For those who could not speak English, their strategies of survival in Chinese catering jobs were to limit their contact with other workers, which did not help in rebuilding connectedness.

Thus, discrimination associated with ableism and sanism worsened their chances in an already unequal labour market offering exploitative working conditions, preventing them from developing an independent life. Welfare benefits were important in preventing further capabilities loss. However, the working of the benefit system and the dominant discourse of benefit scrounging, hindered the receipt of benefits acting as a springboard or buffer zone in terms of capabilities development. Worry about losing their benefits discouraged participants from trying to overcome the hurdles they encountered in looking for paid work. The benefit scrounging discourse caused psychological harm to some participants, leaving them feeling the burden and need to defend and justify themselves by asserting their abnormal and disabled identities.

Stubbornly strive to be human: how hope is experienced and the role of adaptive preferences

In countering the invalidation and discrimination they faced, participants chose different ways of using, or distancing themselves from illness, disabled or service user identities as life strategies. While these identities might help them in asserting a space for existence in the face of a sense of entrapment, they also shaped or restricted how they envisioned their chances for the future. Participants adapted their life goals according to the perceived chances they had as they made sense of the structural barriers they encountered. They also carefully gauged their life plans according to their daily functioning and persisting symptoms, as well as the way they took up or rejected illness, disabled and service users identities.

In this context, I analysed the ways participants experienced hope. The emphasis on hope in the recovery approach rightly stresses the importance of a humanistic orientation in igniting and nurturing users' capacity to aspire (Deegan, 1996a). However, in practice, the way hope or desire was experienced could be capability diminishing and detrimental in nurturing aspiration. This is illustrated through the findings, which show the ways hope, life goals or valued 'doings and beings' were formed. Gender and ethnic ideologies shaped the content of hope. The felt social distance resulting from social class inequalities and consumerism could be channelled into unrealistic aspirations in terms of a restricted notion of the 'good life'. However, I concluded the data analysis on a positive note with examples from participants' narratives showing aspiration for a meaningful life and enhanced agency in the face of restrictive predicaments.

Implications for policy and practice

Policy and service implications concerning mental health policy and services in general, as well as ethnic minorities and Chinese service users in particular can be drawn from this study. The sample size of this study is relatively small because of the formidable challenges encountered during the recruitment phase, as described in the Epilogue. Yet the rich data and valuable insights drawn from the lived experience of the participants proves the importance of documenting and researching the different aspects of Chinese service users' experience. The iatrogenic characteristics of the mental health services, insensitivity to personal needs, paternalistic attitudes of professionals, lack of attention to the meaning attached by the service users, insufficient emphasis on tackling the social determinants of mental distress and ill health, the lack of access to psychological services and the lack of support for independent living are shared criticisms raised by the service user movement. For services to be sensitive to personal needs and socio-economic and cultural circumstances, the research demonstrates the potential of combining the Capabilities Approach with Intersectionality Analysis as an evaluation tool for the recovery process, in order to identify and overcome barriers for the capabilities development of the service users. It can be used in case management for practitioners to assess the needs of the service users. The Capabilities Approach focuses on what exercisable opportunities one has in achieving desired ways of life, rather than what life the person ultimately chooses to live. Thus a Capabilities Approach informed support for service users would steer away from forcing a top-down and narrowly defined recovery goal, such as the 'back to employment', which has been the dominant discourse since the New Labour 'workfare' policies in the UK context, and solicit their valued capabilities from the bottom-up (Ware *et al.*, 2007, 2008; Sacchetto *et al.*, 2016; Tang, 2016). At a community and policy level, the Capabilities Approach can link mental health recovery with actions to discover and tackle the social determinants of (mental) health inequalities, which has gained recognition at the international level (exemplified by the publication of the first report of the Commission on Social Determinants of Health, WHO, in 2008) (Marmot, 2010) but needs to be localised and implemented in the UK (British Academy, 2014). For enhancing mental well-being and facilitating recovery in the community, a transformative community development approach, rather than individualistic intervention, is needed to empower and emancipate service users from the deleterious social inequalities (Tang, 2016).

During the course of this research, the UK underwent significant political and economic changes, which saw the increasing implementation of neo-liberal agendas as well as worsening social inequalities. Some findings of this study served as a testimonial to the detrimental effects of these neo-liberal policies. Participants who have used services for a long time felt acutely aware of the social excluding effect of cuts in funding and services that had been found useful and important for them. The weight of demeaning 'benefit scrounger' discourses on people who claim disability-related benefits were also noticeable in this study. These problems were only exacerbated under the 'austerity' policies pursued by the UK Coalition government after 2010 (Mattheys, 2015). For example, Work Capability Assessment, implemented since 2010, imposes stringent eligibility on disabled people who are out of work. The restriction of benefit provision as well as the assessment process create capabilities deprivation: poverty and worsening mental health (Barr *et al.* 2016). This points to the need for service users of all groups and ethnic identities to defend provision against further cuts in funding and services.

While a cultural explanation may induce victim blaming on individual immigrants and ethnic minorities for 'unsuccessful' acculturation and adaptation to mainstream society and its values (Viruell-Fuentes *et al.*, 2012), a focus on intersecting structural inequalities, as this study has shown, sheds light on how factors such as immigrant policies, labour market and marriage institutions shape behaviours and mental health status. The social conditions portrayed in this study refute the prevalent view common in the UK (and other countries such as the US) that Chinese people as a 'model minority' community is self-contained and can cope by themselves. Thus a general point could be made about this 'model minority' discourse that affects Chinese communities (and other 'model minority' groups such as Japanese, Korean and South Asian communities in the US context). It may serve to legitimise the structural inequalities by encouraging individualised coping skills that are limited in nurturing mental health as shown in this study.

The Intersectionality lens advocated in this research can be incorporated in the cultural competency training of mental health professionals. This can enable health workers to develop holistic ways of understanding the needs of Chinese people (as well as other ethnic minorities) as not only a question of cultural difference, but one that intersects with class, gender and other inequalities (Tang, forthcoming). Furthermore, this study contributed new knowledge on the experience of Chinese ethnic minorities and their mental health (recovery). The social conditions depicted in this research can sensitise policy makers and practitioners in understanding the social causes contributing to their distress and ill health and obstacles for (re) developing capabilities. In the following section, I will highlight parameters for improving health and social care services as well as community development and policies to increase the capabilities of Chinese communities as a whole.

In terms of mental health services, this study echoes other existing literature on Chinese people on the need for better interpretation services and medical pluralism (e.g., Green *et al.* 2002, 2006; Yeung *et al.* 2015). Encouraging and facilitating the transnational usage of health care services *in conjunction with* improving access to local health services can rectify their deprived capability in help-seeking, especially for migrants with low English language capabilities. The stories of the participants illustrated their striving for agency and for recognition of their views while using services. This counters the assumption that Chinese people are compliant and suggests the importance for the health care workers to ask and collaborate with them instead of assuming what they need.

As for community work, findings contradict assumptions of universally harmonious and supportive family and social networks within Chinese communities. This study added further evidence concerning the isolation faced by Chinese elders documented in existing literature (e.g. Tran *et al.* 2008). Service users often strive for independence and the process can involve tension with family members who can be overprotective, or with parents who themselves lack the resources and support. The latter is most apparent for parents who are themselves working-class migrants. Thus, capabilities development for these families as a whole can help them cope with the challenges faced in settling in the UK as well as tackling family problems. Similarly, there is also work to be done in the empowerment of women. Improved mental well-being of women participants in this study were shown alongside their increased capabilities in terms of psychological resources through counselling and economic independence through paid work. However, the gendered division of labour and the reliance on women doing family caring work are still sources of stress for Chinese women that need to be tackled and understood.

Restricted capabilities related to work and employment were especially hard to recover from and develop because of racial discrimination as well as mental health/disability discrimination. This suggests the need for trade unions to reach out to Chinese people as well as mental health service users to provide information as well as support. This also raises the questions whether the mainstream trade unions are equipped to address diversity and equality among their members. The trap of exploitative employment in the Chinese catering business was particularly severe for Chinese people lacking English language skills. Poor working conditions were a cause for mental ill health and the strong stigmatisation in this sector made Chinese service users suffer in silence. As advocated by Kagan *et al.* (2011), enforcement of business, employment and health and safety legislation is needed in this sector. Added to this would be the enforcement of Equality Act and providing information on the discrimination legislations to the workers. Improving working conditions, integrating family-friendly policies as well as mental well-being promotion in this sector would require engagement of Chinese community organisations as well as Chinese businesses.

Conclusions: towards a social justice agenda

Through the study of an ethnic minority community, this book illustrated that inequalities impact on the recovery journeys of service users: from the way inequalities contribute to mental ill health and distress, through the use of mental health services, to their quests in rebuilding a life after crisis and their future outlook. Challenges service users encountered in their recovery were closely linked to intersecting social inequalities. Therefore, this study calls for a social justice agenda for mental health (Harper and Speed, 2012; Morrow and Wessier, 2012; Menzies *et al.*, 2013; Recovery in the Bin, 2016). A social justice agenda would entail a critical examination of the social conditions of causation and evaluation (Pilgrim, 2016), i.e. how class, gender and ethnic inequalities contribute to mental health problems and how ableism and sanism shape the way suffering and madness are contained in the wider socio-economic and political contexts. Mental health policies, adopting the rhetoric of recovery or not, should move from a fixation on rectifying individual pathology to adopt a human rights-based approach in tackling these oppressing structural inequalities. Insights need to be drawn from the lived experiences of service users and their experiential knowledge as demonstrated in this study.

Methodological epilogue
Developing the service user knowledge of Chinese communities

Introduction

In this epilogue, I will explain my research design, a design sought to link micro individual life histories to macro social structures, and reflect on my decisions and challenges encountered during the fieldwork process in relation to the development of service user knowledge of Chinese communities. I will first elaborate on my rationale for using life history as the primary method of addressing the research questions and making links with my theoretical frameworks. Contextualising individuals' recovery journeys in their life courses and social history provides an entry point to analysing the role structural factors play in shaping recovery journeys. The rest of the research design is then discussed and linked with my own experience as a service user located in my translocational positionality.

Next, the uniqueness of user research, the scope of translocational data, the use of purposive sampling and the choice I made to include myself as one of the participants will be addressed. Then I will outline the interview strategies and fieldwork processes and explain the way the fieldwork plan was revised during the fieldwork process. The issues of language, translation and ethics that informed my ideas about making the research process comfortable and empowering for participants, are considered along with my reasons for recruiting participants through Chinese community centres. How the data was thematically analysed in this study will be discussed. This epilogue ends with a reflection on the challenges that were encountered in fieldwork in relation to the collective capability of Chinese communities to nurture and develop service user knowledge.

Life history interview: agency, social location and social structure

I used life history interviewing as a method because it addresses the temporal dimension of recovery journeys and generates information about the social contexts of participants. Experiences of acute periods of mental ill health or crises are a kind of biographical disruption (Bury, 1982; Cardano, 2010), akin to the metaphor of 'shipwreck' in the Tidal Model. Contextualising the recovery journey in one's life course is to explore what has been lost and which aspects of their lives service users strive to 'reclaim', i.e. to 'recover from' (Barker and Buchanan-Baker, 2005: 211). It sheds light on the turning points in the pathway (Elder *et al.*, 2003), through which we can evaluate the process and opportunities dimension of an individual's capabilities development. The turning points that are focused on in this study are the events or processes that led individuals to distress and ill health, how they became psychiatric patients and tried to rebuild their lives after their 'shipwreck'. Asking participants about their choices and decision-making processes at such turning points generates data about what options were available or unavailable to them. This provides an entry point to interpret and analyse exercisable opportunities and explore the interplay of agency and structure. As Bertaux (2003: 40) states,

> Life stories as stories of practices, in which people can describe how they hit these invisible lines, how these lines prevented them from doing what they wanted to do or, on the contrary provided them with unexpected resources, provide a methodological answer to the problem.

The problem Bertaux refers to is how social forces shape social-historical processes and individual life courses. Comparing various life stories in a social-historical context can help in recognising and delineating the invisible workings within and across social relations and institutions. How social structures shape recovery journeys may or may not be consciously known by those recounting their life stories, for the narrative is also conditioned by the social structure (Steensen 2006), resulting in adaptive preferences that limit instead of expanding individuals' capabilities to live a valued life (Sen, 1999; Nussbaum, 2000; Khader, 2011). Therefore, the use of the life history method enables research to take into account the ways an individual's outlook on life change as a result of their perceptions of the limitations they encounter through recovery journey and life course.

As Chapter 2 established, the social location in which the individual is situated is where the interplay of structure and agency is revealed and can be studied. Life history interviewing provides data on the social locations of service users, i.e. how an individual is positioned within a matrix of power relations and social hierarchies formed across history and geographical spaces. The five principles of life history research suggested by Elder *et al.* (2003: 11–14) can help sensitise researchers to how the data generated through biographical interviewing can be used to interpret the positionality of participants.

First, 'the principle of life-span development' suggests that human development and ageing are lifelong processes. It is important to look at how traumas and hardship in childhood impact on an individual's development in adult life (George, 2007), or how deprivation in childhood affects one's biological development and subsequent social pathways resulting in patterns of health inequalities (Wadsworth, 1997). Information about one's formative years can provide insight into how individuals inhabit a social location later in their adult life. Similar to the ethos of the recovery approach, life course research is based on the assumption that human lives can have fundamental and meaningful changes in adulthood. Human beings do not cease to experience significant personal transformations after the adolescent phase. A mental health crisis is sometimes considered as an opportunity to review one's life and to venture into new directions. Therefore, important areas of exploration are what social conditions enable positive changes in terms of the expansion of an individual's capabilities set to address their deprivation in formative years.

Second, 'the principle of agency' stresses how individuals are not the passive agents of social forces. This echoes the theoretical orientation discussed in Chapter 2. The actions of agency can be shown through decision-making processes and turning points at different stages of the recovery journey. For example, the beginning of experiencing distress, medical encounters, getting back to work or study, marital decisions as well as decisions about whether to disclose a mental health history. All these events can provide ideas about what strategies to employ, resources that are available and the constraints faced. All these reflect an individual's capabilities set, which relates to their positionality.

The third and fourth principles link life history interviews with Intersectionality Analysis at the level of the social structure. 'The principle of time and place' emphasises that one's life course is embedded and shaped over a lifetime by historical time and place. Tracing how social history informs a recovery journey and life course is important to understanding the exercisable opportunities in an individual's social location. Relevant data includes the historical events that prompt migration, the economic climate, the labour market, immigration policies and mental health and anti-discrimination legislation. The fourth principle, 'the principle of timing' links to age and normative life course: it is a disciplining dimension intersecting with other inequalities. It seems to be the case that the development of life transitions and related events vary according to their timing in an individual's biography. Elder *et al.* (2003) used a mental health example to illustrate this principle. Quoting Harley and Mortimer (2000) about transition from adolescent to early adulthood, individuals going through a 'pile up' of transitions (e.g. marriage, working life, parenting) had poorer mental health. This illustrates the impact of differing socio-economic status on mental health and the cumulative aspects of differing (dis)advantages.

Looking at the timing or the chronology of life events aids the exploration of the social factors that contribute to mental ill health and recovery. Attention to life stages can also illustrate how intersectionality contributes to the social construction of the normative life course and its effect on agency. Heinz and Kruger (2001) discuss the 'structuration of life course' (p. 36) and the role of institutional arrangements (e.g. welfare regimes, labour markets) on regulation and selection in the life course. The sense of responsibility and expectation of achievement for a given life stage is influenced by culture. For example, gender contributes to such institutional arrangements through cultural concepts of motherhood and domesticity as well as material arrangements reflecting the availability of affordable childcare. The legal pensionable age determined by policy has an influence on how working lives are planned.

The normative life course can have a capability diminishing effect. Shiner *et al.* (2009) argue that a gendered life course perspective offers a better explanation of the relationship between suicide and social bonds than a cruder explanation using social integration because social contact is not necessarily a protective factor when relationships are a source of strain rather than support. The way life course is gendered varies across different ethnic cultures. One may encounter different disciplining forces of normative life course within ethnic communities as well as wider society. In addition, paying attention to the timing of when biographical disruption happens in various life stages can help explore how biographical disruption causes capability deprivation (S.J. Williams, 2000). Such biographical disruption, as a result of mental ill health, may change the social locations one is positioned in along the recovery journey.

Finally, 'the principle of linked lives' points to the interdependence of lived lives and the way socio-historical influences impact on relationships. This generates data about social locations at the level of social relationships, showing how different power relations intersect. The types of relationships here include family relations, intergenerational relations and social networks. One example is the influence of parental well-being on the development of children. The differences and potential conflict of different generations' aspirations is well documented in migration literature (e.g. Dugsin, 2001). Social networks are changed with an individual's geographical movement across and within countries. Asking service users about how their lives are linked to significant others as well as wider social networks can generate data about the power relations they are in and how their worldviews, life aspirations and recovery goals have been shaped in relation to significant others. In this study, the relationship between mental health professionals and service users are viewed as important in influencing the support received from service providers. The power of mental health professionals is sanctioned through mental health legislation. Therefore this study explored how the matrix of power relations embedded in social locations can generate data about the extent to which individuals exercise agency and utilise these relations in realising a meaningful recovery.

The social location of the researcher: service user knowledge, translocational data and purposive sampling

It is not only the life stories of participants that have contributed to this study. Mills (2000) argues that sociological works, and intellectual works in general, are inseparable from researchers' own biographies and life experiences. The past influences a researcher's orientation and decisions about their current work, just as the history of service users impact on their current plans and outlook on recovery. So it is important for researchers to reflect on how their life experiences knowingly, or inadvertently, guide the research process. In the following section I will consider the impact of my past experiences and social locations on my research design. The decisions I made about its focus on service user experience and knowledge, the fine-tuning of the life history interviewing with its emphasis on translocational dimension, and finally, purposive sampling including the use of myself as one of the participants will be elaborated.

More than about 'voices': user researcher and service user generated knowledge

Critical voices and knowledge generated from the lived experience of service users are important to understanding metal health and its recovery (Faulkner, 2004). Proponents of narrative therapy suggest that service users can find telling their own stories is therapeutic, empowering and may contribute to them constructing a positive sense of self (Semmler and Williams, 2000). Yet the importance of building experiential knowledge is more than 'giving service users a voice'. It is also about challenging and building knowledge about mental health in general and informing service users, carers and professionals about strategies for recovery and/or survival (Russo and Sweeney, 2016). Mental health is a contested field of study and so the experiential knowledge of service users should not be neglected. As Rose puts it, 'psychiatry deals in human matters. Should it not then pay attention to the worlds of meaning that its patients inhabit? Yet it regularly does not do this' (2009: 41).

There are questions that cannot be researched using randomised controlled trials (the 'gold standard' of scientific study) alone. For example, questions such as why service users choose one treatment instead of another can only be answered through studying personal experience and the meanings embedded in decision-making processes. If the recovery approach is to move beyond symptom relief and ensure a quality of life, then recovery research must explore relevant aspects of service users' lives and how they impact on the treatments and strategies service users utilise to survive. This means that qualitative research about subjective lived experience is critical to answering such questions. Research questions formed by users, inspired from their own experiences, can address important areas that professionals may fail to attend to. This research study is one such example.

My personal experience as a mental health service user inspired my interest in research about the way the recovery approach is being mainstreamed in mental health policy and the choice to focus on Chinese service users in the UK. I was born and grew up in Hong Kong during its colonial era and then lived in the UK for 7 years. My history of using mental health services began when I was in Hong Kong, and I accessed public psychiatric services in the UK. I underwent different kinds of treatment including medications and psychological therapies, and consider myself recovered now. My interest in mental health was formed after a major breakdown during my mid-twenties. It was a biographical disruption for me; it felt like a shipwreck and emerging from it I started to feel that mental illness had left its mark on my orientation to life and what life meant to me. Mental illness became something big in my life, in the sense that when I made decisions about the future I found mental illness to be a weight on my shoulder that I could not shrug off. It was about coping with existing symptoms, worrying about relapses and stigma and something more.

After coming to the UK and encountering the service user movement I started to reflect on and articulate about what the weight I carried meant. Having the space to consider my positive and negative service experiences, including the process of treatment, was important. This space was, in my experience, limited if not totally absent in Hong Kong. The dominance of bio-medical professionalism somehow subsumed my negative experiences of being treated in the psychiatric system. While I was being treated in Hong Kong I found that I had to give up agency in exchange for care. There were rules and hidden scripts that I had to follow. Deviance from these rules was considered to be a symptom of abnormality. When I came to the UK and made contact with the service users movement I realised I had become an 'insider' of the mental health world. This gave me the insight that what service users recover from could include mental health service encounters. The feeling of powerlessness in the face of the power inequality between professionals and service users was expressed in ways that were heavy-handed, if not human rights violations. I met good professionals and had useful treatments that I deeply appreciated. However, there were also invalidations and ridiculous incidents that happened to me and other service users. For me, the power of service user research comes from reflection on the good and bad and the development of informed alternatives about what helps different service users to pursue their unique recovery journeys.

Apart from the generation of research questions from a service user standpoint, the distinctiveness of service user research can also be found in other parts of the research process that inform this study. In terms of data collection, it has been found that research which involved service users as interviewers, generated more open and honest responses from interviewees (e.g. Rose, 2001; Allam *et al.*, 2004). In relation to data interpretation, the contribution of service users' experiential knowledge has the potential of producing well-rounded and detailed work. This is because experiential knowledge is embodied in the user researcher 'having the knowledge of the sensations, depths of feelings and meanings, and the abject horrors of how illness can impact on one's life' (Straughan, 2009: 115). Thus emotionality can be put to positive use in the research process, instead of being viewed, as it is by positivist researchers, as an obstacle.

I considered different ways of increasing the level of user involvement in this study. There are different models of service user involvement in research in terms of the research stages they participate in, for example, an individual study or participatory action research (Wallcraft and Nettle, 2009). Because of the time and resource constraints of a PhD study, I did not employ a more participatory model of research. I considered setting up an advisory group formed by Chinese service users alongside a mental health project that the first Chinese community centre I contacted planned to run. However the Centre did not secure funding for the project so I could not go ahead with this plan. I decided to run a focus group as both a preparation for the in-depth interviews and to explore the possibility of forming an advisory group. However, the focus group did not take place as some of the participants could not attend because of their persisting and fluctuating symptoms. Therefore, I decided to carry out individual in-depth interviews as the primary data collection method.

Differences, researcher's positionality and translocational life history

I share some commonalities with other mental health service users, which made it easier for me to gain the trust of participants and understand what questions to ask. I found the critiques of the UK service user movement resonated with my experiences. However, I was aware of how my social location could have made a difference to the path my recovery journey took compared with other people. Thinking about possible commonalities and differences increased my determination to collect data that captured the diversity of participant's experiences. First, there is the discrimination I experienced as a Chinese migrant and member of an ethnic minority. This experience was harmful to my mental well-being but was not something that my British service user friends could easily identify with. Second, there are differences, often privileges, which I have compared with other immigrants from China or Hong Kong. My university qualification and research training in Hong Kong were transferrable skills that I used to find employment in the UK mainstream labour market. I had more choices in seeking support as I could access mainstream voluntary services with my English language capability. Having worked alongside other mental health professionals, educators and service users, I developed a social network that I could draw upon during a relapse. Reflecting on these privileges, I was aware of the different challenges service users face because of unequal capabilities sets, resulting from different ethnicity, class background, gender and age.

Living in both Hong Kong and the UK, and having some understanding of the context of mainland China through my family network, enabled me to be sensitive to structural level differences such as health care systems, labour markets and other social institutions that constitute the different barriers service users encounter. This diversity of experience needed to be understood in a transnational context. To capture and understand the structural factors contributing to the variations in the recovery journeys of Chinese service users in the UK, the life history interviews I carried out paid attention to translocational dimensions. Contextualising recovery journeys through life histories is to take a holistic view of an individual's struggle. As I mentioned in Chapter 2, such contextualisation would not be sufficiently deep for a study of members of an ethnic minority if it did not take the translocational dimensions of life histories into account. What I call 'translocational life history', looks at inequalities of class, gender and ethnicity not only at a national (UK) level, but also in relation to the home countries of migrants as well as inequalities at a transnational level. Migration history and experiences of distress and using mental health services in home countries were essential to my research focus. In addition 'translocational life history' is relevant to British-born Chinese participants, because their parents or grandparents immigrated from another country and are likely to maintain contact with relatives and families there. This group could be influenced by Chinese cultures e.g. the proliferation of popular culture facilitated by media, which prompted my enquiry into transnational social networks and senses of belonging and identity.

Purposive sampling and use of self as a participant

I decided to include myself as one of the participants. It was a decision made at a late stage of the fieldwork. One of the participants asked me why I did not include my own experiences in the study. My immediate reaction was that it was not a usual academic research practice, and this project has to fulfil the criteria for a PhD thesis. The concerns I had at first were methodological. I felt that I had to maintain the role of a 'distant' interpreter. Interpreting my own experiences would mean that I would be too 'close' to the data and might lose sight of the meanings emerging from it. Also I had to ensure that the data was collected consistently from all participants. Interviewing myself or talking into a recorder would make the data collection inconsistent. Moreover, I worried that since I already had a voice as an interpreter and narrator of the biographies, my presence might become too 'dominating' in the study. I thought that the place of a researcher's own experience should be confined to the reflexive account in the methodology chapter.

However, my aim was to research Chinese service users' experiences in the UK partly because this group was under-represented within the mainstream mental health literature, and I discovered it was not easy to collect Chinese service users' narratives in an in-depth way as will be discussed later. So it seems to be a 'waste' not to include my own experience too. To reconcile these methodological concerns, I decided that I could still follow the data collection method I had set up for the rest of the participants, if I asked a trusted friend who had research experience to interview me. I familiarised my friend with the research objectives and interview guide I had designed. I, like the other participants, could decide how much I wanted to reveal. The interview was recorded and transcribed like the other interviews. I gave myself a pseudonym and treated myself as one of a set of life histories cases during the analysis stage. Being interviewed, transcribing my interview and assigning myself a pseudonym worked well as devices that helped me to defamiliarise myself from my raw experiences.

Language, translations, ethics and access

Preparation for fieldwork also included language and translation issues relevant to the data collection. Publicity, an introduction to the research and a consent form were produced in two sets of bilingual language, one with simplified Chinese and English and the other with traditional Chinese and English. This was designed to cater for the language diversity within Chinese communities, as people from Hong Kong use traditional Chinese characters while those from mainland China used simplified Chinese for written text.

Slade *et al.* (2012) raise the issue of the translatability of Western concepts in non-Western worlds. Their review of publications in 11 Western and non-Western countries, found that the conceptualisation of recovery in these countries was largely the same, covering 'connectedness', 'hope and optimism', 'identity', 'meaning in life' and 'empowerment'. While this might mean that the Western conceptualisation of recovery in the recovery movement was being increasingly recognised in non-Western countries, Slade *et al.* (2012) suggest that that recovery-related concepts already existed in non-Western cultures. These concepts reflect worldviews that differ from those of Western cultures, such as an emphasis on the relationship of human beings to the physical world or an emphasis on body, spirit and mind in conceptualisations of identity and health. In the Chinese language, 復元/圓/原 (*Fu Yuan*) is commonly used when denoting 'recovery'. The first means 'regaining vitality and life force', the second means 'regaining fullness and completeness' while the third implies a restoration to an original state (Tse *et al.*, 2012: 44).

Another recovery-related concept 'wellness' also raised the issues of translatability. I discussed the translation of the word 'wellness' with a Chinese community worker when a community centre was considering providing 'WRAP' (Wellness Recovery Action Plan) training. We struggled to find a directly equivalent concept in the Chinese language. In recent years, the word '幸福感' (*xing fu gan*) has been used increasingly in the mass media and academy of mainland China and Hong Kong when surveys or indexes of wellness are referred to. '幸福感' (*xing fu gan*) comes close to the meaning of 'wellness' as it captures the non-health aspect of 'well-being', subjective preferences about life directions, as well as having a meaning larger than 'subjective happiness'. Yet I felt that something was being lost in the translation. In the information about my research that I designed for participants, I used '康復' (*kang fu*) instead as it was the aim of the research to elicit the different subjective understandings and worldviews of the participants, which were then used to interrogate the mainstream meaning of 'recovery' discourse in mental health services in the UK, Hong Kong and mainland China. Therefore, I used the word '*kang fu*' in the written material as well as during the interview.

I gave a lot of consideration to ensuring that participants felt comfortable and safe while being interviewed. With the help of Chinese community centres, I was able to book rooms in their premises where the participants could choose to be interviewed. They could also choose to meet elsewhere. For example, I met participants in cafes or their homes. This flexibility about meeting places was important. One participant disliked going to public places. Another preferred to stay at home because she was struggling with fluctuating symptoms and could find travelling difficult. One was concerned about stigma. So he asked to be interviewed in a Western-style restaurant as he thought he would not be 'found out' by his friend or other Chinese people, on whom he relied for employment. When I asked him what diagnosis he had received, he chose to write it down on paper instead of telling me, worrying that people in the cafe might eavesdrop.

Life story reminiscence can be cathartic for interviewees (Dickson-Swift *et al.*, 2007). It can also be distressing when it involves recounting painful experiences. Becoming a participant in this kind of research can be an important part of the recovery process for some service users (Hamilton, 2009). For this reason, I asked about the support and the services provided by Chinese community centres and I established with community centre staff that participants might need to use these after their interviews. I explained to participants that research was not a counselling service. If they needed support, they could ask for it from staff in the centres.

Procedures about confidentially were also followed and detailed in written form. Participants could choose not to be tape-recorded. One participant chose this as she worried that her complaints during the interview might trigger retaliation. I also told the participants that pseudonyms would be used in the research write-up to protect their identity. In this book, pseudonyms are used throughout except for one person. Raymond preferred to use his real name as he thought he had nothing to hide or feel ashamed of. His viewpoint was a good reminder of what a service user friend had said to me about service user involvement in research during a workshop. For mental health service users who had experiences of being pathologised in scientific research, having a choice to disclose themselves, for example, by using their real names in research, was a way for them to positively assert their identity.

I also considered ways that participants might find being interviewed a meaningful and empowering process. One in which they would feel they were treated with respect and equality. I was open to participants about my use of mental health services and shared my experiences if they asked about them. At the end of each interview, I would ask if there was anything else they wanted to ask me about the research or other things. Some participants asked about my experiences and we shared information about the difficulties we had experienced and how we had coped with them. I cannot speak for the participants, but for me the exchanges were empowering because I felt empathy. This empathy came from mutual understanding of how hard it is to live and deal with mental health problems. I hoped the participants felt the same.

Some participants saw me as a mental health professional who might be able to offer counselling or other services. In order not to raise false hopes I made it clear that I was not in the position to do this and gave them information about services that I knew about. In order to place value on their time and knowledge, participants were given a sum of £15 as an honorarium, which also covered their travel expenses. The sum was determined by three considerations. First, thanks to external funding, I was able to pay more than travel expenses to the participants. Second, I wanted to place value on their expertise and knowledge as 'experts by experience', a term that stresses the knowledge gained in having survived the experience (Hamilton, 2009; Wallcraft and Nettle, 2009). Third, people who have received a diagnosis can often experience economic disadvantages as a result of unemployment. The payment I made was designed to enhance the value of the process and outcomes of my research as well as providing participants with an experience that placed value on their expertise and knowledge.

Access and recruitment

Participants were recruited through community organisations serving Chinese communities rather than the National Health Service (NHS). As discussed previously, the nature of the interviews involved probing into a lot of personal, and sometimes painful, experiences. Participants need to be able to build trust and feel confident with the interviewer. I contacted the staff of Chinese community organisations, explained the rationale of the research and my own background, and asked if they could help me to publicise the research project and introduce potential participants to it. If the participants expressed doubts about the project and being interviewed, not only could they contact me directly but they could also talk to the staff they were acquainted with. If participants had been recruited by letter via the NHS, they might not be have been able to get a second opinion from staff about whether or not to take part. The help of the community centres also meant that participants could choose to be interviewed in a familiar community centre. Participants were, in the main, recruited through Chinese community organisations in Birmingham, Manchester and London. The original plan was to focus on one city and to conduct recruitment as part of the development of a mental health project with Birmingham Chinese Community Centre as already mentioned. I also promoted the research through Chinese-speaking private doctors and churches for Chinese people, as these are two locations used by members of Chinese communities.

In the early phase of the fieldwork, I planned to focus on a single city. As the configuration of the NHS varies in different regions, I hoped that focus on a single city could give in-depth contextual information about the local set up of the health and social care provision. It was also easier to recruit a sufficient sample in a big city than in rural areas because of the concentration of Chinese communities in such cities. Although London has a large Chinese community, there have been several studies of Chinese people's health there because there are national as well as local Chinese associations based in the capital. Birmingham is the UK's second largest city. It has a prominent Chinese population but the mental health services provided by Chinese community centres there were still developing. This meant that my research findings might have been helpful to Chinese communities in Birmingham. Nevertheless I found that I was not able to recruit enough participants in Birmingham for reasons that I will explain later. Because of the time constraints on my PhD, I decided to trade off the collection of embedded local data for feasibility. I revised my recruitment strategies and recruited participants in two other cities, London and Manchester, with the help of two local, established Chinese community centres. A total of 22 participants were recruited (including myself). The recruitment stopped when I became aware of redundancy in the accounts within the emerging themes.

Data analysis

The interpretation of the social locations was carried out during each interview to make sense of the participants' recovery journey. Interviews were transcribed verbatim and were coded with the following codes: diagnosis and nature of distress, migration experience, types of health and social service used, living conditions such as types of housing, work history and working conditions, domestic life, types of benefits received if any, as well as the main themes brought up in the interviews. Emerging themes were then developed from these codes. Under each theme, participants were compared and contrasted according to their different social locations. Themes were structured around organisational, institutional, discursive, experiential or social interactional 'societal arenas' as proposed by Anthias for intersectionality studies (1998, 2013). Capabilities changes, i.e. what and how capabilities were expanded or contracted, are the expression of the way the different dimensions of domination and subordination result in reinforcing or contradicting the social locations that service users occupy. Through comparing the experiences and capabilities of service users in similar or different social locations within and across societal arenas, I carried out a close analysis of how different power relations play out in shaping the social conditions that lead to capabilities diminishment or the capability development that is crucial to mental well-being and living a meaningful life.

Challenges and reflections on building a collective capability of knowledge development

As discussed in Chapter 1, this research started with an intention to develop service user knowledge about what works for recovery in Chinese communities. The challenges I encountered during the research process reflect what needs to be in place for Chinese communities to develop a collective capability of knowledge development (Deneulin, 2008). There are three dimensions to this capability development. The first concerns the capability of community organisations. Having to widen points of access in order to recruit enough participants reflected the challenges Chinese community centres faced in developing mental health services in the UK. The Birmingham community centre had run a mental health project with a focus on mental health promotion with a part-time staff member for a few years before my research began. As a linking point through which statutory services sought consultation, good relationships had been developed between the community centre and the city council as well as the local NHS. NHS consultation events had been organised through the centre to increase understanding of Chinese people's needs in the city. Although the centre was keen to develop mental health services once the funding for the project finished, they were not able to secure further funding. This meant that the momentum that had been developed was slowed down because of a lack of resources, e.g. staff time. Resource-strapped staff were less able to support new people who contacted the centre. The experience and knowledge developed through the mental health project could not be sustained because of reduced staff capacity. It is beyond the scope of this research to study the factors that may facilitate or constrain the development of community centers for Chinese communities. Nonetheless, the role of a community centre as a space in which to nurture and consolidate the knowledge base of service users as 'expert by experience' is an important topic for future research.

The capability development of individual service users to reflect on their own experiences is also vital in building a service user knowledge base. As I argued in Chapter 2, knowledge production that starts from a standpoint does not necessarily reflect emancipatory values. Reflexivity marks the difference between a consumerist model of service user involvement in which users' voices are taken at face value and a participatory model in which service users collectively reflect on their own and others' experience to draw out transferable knowledge. In this research, it became clear that in-depth interviews were a reflexivity development process. Yanos and Hopper (2008) drew upon Bourdieu's concept of 'false, collusive objectification' (1999: 616) to discuss interview bias resulting from the performance of interviewees according to their perceived expectation of the interviewers. (This concept is akin to 'adaptive preference' in the Capabilities Approach.)

> [F]alse, because it is unfaithful to the particularities of the life under scrutiny; collusive, because the interviewer unwittingly goes along with the artifice; and objectifying because a readymade account has been substituted for the lived, unfinished angularities of a reflective subject.
>
> (Yanos and Hopper, 2008: 230)

The result is that ambivalence, inconsistencies, and yet-to-be-articulated feelings and dilemmas in authentic experience were subsumed under a narrative that sounds pleasing and familiar to the researcher. Yanos and Hopper argue that this 'false, collusive objectification' is often found in mental health interviews in which service users narrate a 'model' success story with a plot adhering to clinical psychiatric terms such as 'insights' and 'denials'.

During my fieldwork, such 'false, collusive objectification' could be found in some interviews. For example, when I asked participants what advice they would give to other service users, they would sometimes provide me with the 'standard script' of mental health promotion material such as going to the doctor and taking prescribed medication. However, in the same interviews, they talked about concerns, grievances, ambivalence or uncertainties in their past experience of using services or having treatments as well as other ways they successfully managed their stress. I do not mean that this discrepancy implies the latter is necessarily more 'true' than the standard scripts. But if a researcher does not pay attention to discrepancy and complexity and is satisfied with 'standard scripts', they may lose the transformative power that comes from knowledge accumulated from service users' lived experiences. Yanos and Hopper (2008) argue that a reason 'false, collusive objectification' was often found in mental health interview topics could be because this topic relates powerfully to participant's identity. The narration of participants is a way they self-manage their identity.

Yanos and Hopper's reading of Bourdieu offered me realist solutions to enhance the authenticity of the interviews in order to obtain nuanced, complex data about lived experience: active listening, in-depth knowledge of the circumstances relevant to the respondent, repeated interviews, attention to clichés that may reflect the bias of the participants as well as that of the interviewers, a willingness to classify interviews as unusable. In this research, I drew attention to the complexities, ambiguities, and inconsistencies of the stories told by the participants during the interview. This was not about challenging service users' accounts. On the contrary, it was an invitation to participants to go on a reflexive journey in which we could explore together discrepancy and nuance in their accounts. The interview process was thus a co-reflexive process between the researcher and the participant. This process was designed to obtain richer data and make the interview an empowering process that facilitated reflexivity development.

The third dimension for Chinese communities to build service user knowledge is to develop service user researchers, i.e. researchers that openly bring their personal experience to the research process. As I discussed earlier in this chapter, I was careful not to assume that all service users go through the same experiences, hold the same opinions or find that what worked for them worked for others. Reflexivity and respecting varieties of experience are important capabilities for user researchers. The other aspect of developing the capacity of service user research concerns emotionality. While I found that my embodied knowledge of lived experience enhanced the research process and data analysis, the impact of such emotionality on a researcher's well-being cannot be underestimated.

When I decided to actively use my personal experience in this research, I anticipated that it would be an emotional process for me not only because of the emotional impact a qualitative research on a sensitive topic could bring (Dickson-Swift *et al.*, 2008), but also because of my closeness to this research topic. However, the impact was much greater than I anticipated. The impact was apparent throughout the research process, but intensified during the fieldwork stage when the interviews were carried out. Listening to the stories told by the participants triggered memories of my own distress and negative experiences. Sometimes feelings of empathy would lead me to want to help participants although I was also clear that I was not in a position to do this. This left me feeling frustrated and powerless. The fieldwork became a recovery journey for me. The transcription process was difficult too: hearing the recording and verbatim transcribing was like re-living the interview process. Writing up was equally emotionally draining.

While I was determined to see this project through and the rich data collected made me certain about the value of service user research, I realised that it is important to have a support system in place for service user researchers. Faulkner (2004) in her consultation with service user researchers about their experiences of involvement in research came up with guidance about the ethics of service user research. She suggested that emotional support for service user researchers might take the form of peer support or access to a person who is not attached to the project, so that they can focus on emotionally supporting the researcher rather than managing the research. I chose to ask a trusted friend to be a mentor who I met after interviews when I felt the process had been overwhelming. This mentor proved to be important to me in sustaining my emotional well-being as a user researcher.

Enabling the development of service users' experiential knowledge is crucial in expanding the collective capability of Chinese communities. It not only gives voice to a marginalised group, but could also help develop agendas for change set by communities at the local level (Kalathil et al., 2011b). The three dimensions I discussed suggest support needed at the institutional and individual levels. The way recovery approach and user involvement were mainstreamed by the mental health system were disputed by activists; they argue that recovery and user movement were coopted by neo-liberal mental health policies that individualise personal distress and render user participation tokenistic (Beresford, 2016). Thus to regain their emancipatory potentials as originally advocated by service users, reasserting the significance of service user generated knowledge (Russo and Sweeney, 2016) and a continuous exploration of good practices in supporting co-production of knowledge (Carr and Patel, 2016) are central to a social justice agenda that challenges inequalities, including the inequalities in knowledge production, to transform mental health policies and practices (Carr and Patel, 2016; Russo and Sweeney, 2016).

Appendix

Participants' biographical data

	Name	Gender	Age	Place of origin
1	Abao	F	53	Mainland China
2	Bai-Xin	F	55	Mainland China
3	Carol	F	38	Hong Kong
4	Danny	M	42	Hong Kong
5	Eric	M	25	Hong Kong
6	Feng	M	28	Mainland China
7	Hins	F	31	Mainland China
8	In-Lei	F	70	Mainland China
9	Jerry	M	41	UK
10	Ken	M	45	Hong Kong
11	Lai-Ming	M	65	Hong Kong
12	Marcus	M	65	Hong Kong
13	Nin-Jin	F	51	Hong Kong
14	Oa-Yang	F	64	Hong Kong
15	Pun-Yi	F	58	Hong Kong
16	Rachel	F	31	Vietnam
17	Raymond	M	27	UK
18	Shun-Tien	F	82	Hong Kong
19	Tang-Yung	F	43	Mainland China
20	Wu-Wei	F	31	Mainland China
21	Young	M	33	Hong Kong
22	Zoie	F	31	Hong Kong

References

Adamson, S. *et al.* 2009. *Hidden from public view? Racism against the UK's Chinese population.* London: The Monitoring Group. Online. Available at www.sociology. leeds.ac.uk/assets/files/research/cers/Min%20Quan%20Finished%20Report.pdf (accessed 31 October 2016).

Ahmad, W.I.U. and Atkin, K. (eds) 1996. *'Race' and community care.* Buckingham: Open University Press.

Allam, S. *et al.* 2004. 'Our experience of collaborative research: service users, carers and researchers work together to evaluate an assertive outreach service'. *Journal of Psychiatric and Mental Health Nursing* 11 (3): 368–373.

Allott, P., Loganathan, L. and Fulford, K.W.M. 2002. 'Discovering hope for recovery: a review of a selection of recovery literature, implications for practice and systems change'. *Canadian Journal of Community Mental Health* 21 (2): 13–33.

Anthias, F. 1998. 'Rethinking social divisions: some notes towards a theoretical framework'. *The Sociological Review* 46 (3): 505–535.

Anthias, F. 2001. 'New hybridities, old concepts: the limits of culture'. *Ethnic and Racial Studies* 24 (4): 619–641.

Anthias, F. 2006. 'Belongings in a globalising and unequal world: rethinking translocations'. In N. Yuval-Davis, K. Kannabirān and U. Vieten (eds) *The situated politics of belonging.* London: Sage, pp. 17–31.

Anthias, F. 2013. 'Intersectional what? Social divisions, intersectionality and levels of analysis'. *Ethnicities* 13 (1): 3–19.

Anthony, W.A. 1993. 'Recovery from mental illness: the guiding vision of the mental health service system in the 1990s'. *Psychosocial Rehabilitation Journal* 16 (4): 11–23.

Archer, L. and Francis, B. 2005. '"They never go off the rails like other ethnic groups": teachers' constructions of British Chinese pupils' gender identities and approaches to learning'. *British Journal of Sociology of Education* 26 (2): 165–182.

Archer, L. and Francis, B. 2006. *Understanding minority ethnic achievement: race, gender, class and 'success'.* Abingdon, UK: Routledge.

Archer, M.S. 2000. *Being human: the problem of agency.* Cambridge: Cambridge University Press.

Ariana, P. and Naveed, A. 2009. 'Health'. In S. Denenulin and L. Shahani (eds) *An introduction to the human development and capability approach: freedom and agency.* London: Earthscan, pp. 229–245.

Armour, M., Bradshaw, W. and Roseborough, D. 2009. 'African Americans and recovery from severe mental illness'. *Social Work in Mental Health* 7 (6): 602–622.

Armstrong, D. 1994. *Outline of sociology as applied to medicine*. 4th edn. Oxford: Butterworth Heinemann.

Arun, S.V., Arun, T.G. and Borooah, V.K. 2004. 'The effect of career breaks on the working lives of women'. *Feminist Economics* 10 (1): 65–84.

Aydinligil, S. 2009. 'Gender policy in Turkey'. In S. Denenulin and L. Shahani (eds) *An introduction to the human development and capability approach: freedom and agency*. London: Earthscan, pp. 304–311.

Balint, M. 1964. *The doctor, his patient and the illness*. 2nd edn. London: Pitman Medical.

Barham, P. and Hayward, R. 1991. *From the mental patient to the person*. London: Routledge.

Barker, P.J. 2003. 'The Tidal Model: psychiatric colonization, recovery and the paradigm shift in mental health care'. *International Journal of Mental Health Nursing* 12 (2): 96–102.

Barker, P.J. and Buchanan-Barker, P. 2005. *The Tidal Model: a guide for mental health professionals*. Hove: Brunner-Routledge.

Barr, B. *et al.* 2016. '"First, do no harm": are disability assessments associated with adverse trends in mental health? A longitudinal ecological study'. *Journal of Epidemiology and Community Health* 70 (4): 339–345.

Barrow, S.M. *et al.*, 2014. 'Context and opportunity: multiple perspectives on parenting by women with a severe mental illness'. *Psychiatric Rehabilitation Journal* 37 (3): 176–182.

Baxter, S.C.C. 1988. *A political economy of the ethnic Chinese catering industry*. PhD Thesis, Aston University. Online. Available at http://eprints.aston.ac.uk/12180/ (accessed 31 October 2016).

BBC. 15 June 2009. 'Council loses £1m sickness case'. Online. Available at http://news.bbc.co.uk/2/hi/uk_news/england/gloucestershire/8100126.stm (accessed 31 October 2016).

Beck, A.T. 1976. *Cognitive therapy and the emotional disorders*. New York: International Universities Press.

Beresford, P. 2000. 'What have madness and psychiatric system survivors got to do with disability and disability studies?' *Disability and Society* 15 (1): 167–172.

Beresford, P. 2002. 'Thinking about "mental health": Towards a social model'. *Journal of Mental Health* 11 (6): 581–584.

Beresford, P. 2016. 'From psycho-politics to mad studies: learning from the legacy of Peter Sedgwick'. *Critical and Radical Social Work* 4 (3): 343–355.

Beresford, P., Nettle, M. and Perring, R. 2012. *Towards a social model of madness and distress: exploring what service users say*. New York: Joseph Rowntree Foundation. Online. Available at www.jrf.org.uk/sites/files/jrf/mental-health-service-models-full.pdf (accessed 30 October 2016)

Bertaux, D. 2003. 'The usefulness of life stories for a realist and meaningful sociology'. In R. Humphrey, R.L. Miller and E.A. Zdravomyslova (eds) *Biographical research in Eastern Europe: altered lives and broken biographies*. Aldershot: Ashgate, pp. 39–52.

Bhaskar, R. 1989. *Reclaiming reality: a critical introduction to contemporary philosophy*. London: Verso.

Borg, M. and Davidson, L. 2008. 'The nature of recovery as lived in everyday experience'. *Journal of Mental Health* 17 (2): 129–140.

Bourdieu, P. 1999. 'Understanding'. In P. Bourdieu *et al.* (eds) *The weight of the world: social suffering in contemporary society*. Cambridge: Polity Press, pp. 607–626.

Boydell, K., Gladstone, B. and Crawford, E. (2002) 'The dialectic of friendship for people with psychiatric disabilities'. *Psychiatric Rehabilitation Journal* 26 (2): 123–131.

Bradley, A. 2006. 'Biographical disruption or reinforcement? Men's life histories of emotional distress'. Unpublished PhD Thesis, University of Warwick. Online. Available at http://wrap.warwick.ac.uk/39836/ (accessed 31 October 2016).

Brown, G. W., Harris, T. O., and Hepworth, C. 1995. 'Loss, humiliation and entrapment among women developing depression: a patient and non-patient comparison'. *Psychological Medicine* 25(1): 7–22.

Bury, M. 1982. 'Chronic illness as biographical disruption'. *Sociology of Health and Illness* 4 (2): 167–182.

Campbell, F.K. 2009. *Contours of ableism*. Basingstoke: Palgrave Macmillan.

Cardano, M. 2010. 'Mental distress: strategies of sense-making'. *Health* 14 (3): 253–271.

Care Quality Commission. 2010. *Count me in 2009: results of the 2009 national census of inpatients and patients on supervised community treatment in mental health and learning disability services in England and Wales*. London: Care Quality Commission. Online. Available at www.cqc.org.uk/sites/default/files/documents/count_me_in_2010_final_tagged.pdf (accessed 31 October 2016).

Care Services Improvement Partnership, Royal College of Psychiatrists and Social Care Institute for Excellence. 2007. *A common purpose: recovery in future mental health services*. SCIE Position Paper 08. London: Social Care Institute for Excellence. Online. Available at www.scie.org.uk/publications/positionpapers/pp08.pdf (accessed 31 October 2016).

Carpenter, M. 2009a. 'A third wave, not a third way? New labour, human rights and mental health in historical context'. *Social Policy and Society* 8 (2): 215–230.

Carpenter, M. 2009b. 'The capabilities approach and critical social policy: Lessons from the majority world?' *Critical Social Policy* 29 (3): 351–373.

Carr, S. and Patel, M. 2016. *Practical guide: progressing transformative co-production in mental health*. Bath: the National Development Team for Inclusion.

Chamberlayne, P., Bornat, J. and Wengraf, T. 2000. 'Introduction: biographical turn'. In Chamberlayne, P., Bornat, J. and Wengraf, T. (eds) *The turn to biographical methods in social science: comparative issues and examples.* London: Routledge, pp. 1–30.

Chamberlin, J. 1978. *On our own: patient-controlled alternatives to the mental health system*. New York: McGraw-Hill.

Chau, R.C.M. 2008. *Health experiences of Chinese people in the UK*. Better Health Briefing Paper 10. London: Race Equality Foundation. Online. Available at www.better-health.org.uk/sites/default/files/briefings/downloads/health-brief10.pdf (accessed 31 October 2016).

Chau, R.C.M. and Yu, S.W.K. 2001. 'Social exclusion of Chinese people in Britain'. *Critical Social Policy* 21 (1): 103–125.

Chau, R.C.M., Yu, S.W.K. and Tran, C.T.L. 2011. 'The diversity based approach to culturally sensitive practices'. *International Social Work* 54 (1): 21–33.

Chau, R.C.M., Yu, S.W.K. and Tran, C.T.L. 2012. 'Understanding the diverse health needs of Chinese people in Britain and developing cultural sensitive services'. *Journal of Social Work* 12 (4): 385–403.

Chinese Society of Psychiatry. 2001. *Chinese classification of mental disorders (CCMD-3)*. 3rd edn. Beijing: Chinese Society of Psychiatry.

Choo, H.Y. and Ferree, M.M. 2010. 'Practicing intersectionality in sociological research: a critical analysis of inclusions, interactions, and institutions in the study of inequalities'. *Sociological Theory* 28 (2): 129–149.

Clark, M. 2007. 'Knitting up the unravelled sleeve: my journey through mental distress to recovery'. Paper presented at the Narrative Practitioner Conference, Glyndŵr University.

Cochrane, R. and Bal, S.S. 1989. 'Mental hospital admission rates of immigrants to England: a comparison of 1971 and 1981'. *Social Psychiatry and Psychiatric Epidemiology* 24: 2–11.

Coleman, R. 2004. *Recovery: an alien concept?* Wormit, Fife: P&P Press.

Collins, P.H. 1998. 'It's all in the family: intersections of gender, race, and nation'. *Hypatia* 13 (3): 62–82.

Commission on Social Determinants of Health 2008. *Closing the gap in a generation: health equity through action on the social determinants of health.* Geneva: World Health Organisation.

Corin, E. and Lauzon, G. 1994. 'From symptoms to phenomena: the articulation of experience in schizophrenia'. *Journal of Phenomenological Psychology* 25 (1): 3–50.

Corrigan, P., Markowitz, F. and Watson, A. (2004) 'Structural levels of mental illness stigma and discrimination'. *Schizophrenia Bulletin* 30 (3): 481–491.

Costa, B. 2013. *Language support: challenges and benefits for users and providers of health and social care services.* Better Health Briefing Paper 26. London: Race Equality Foundation. Online. Available at www.better-health.org.uk/sites/default/files/briefings/downloads/Language%20Support-%20formatted.pdf (accessed 31 October 2016).

Craig, G. and Walker, R. 2012. '"Race" on the welfare margins: the UK government's Delivering Race Equality mental health programme'. *Community Development Journal* 47 (4): 491–505.

Crenshaw, K. 1991. 'Mapping the margins: intersectionality, identity politics, and violence against women of color'. *Stanford Law Review* 43 (6): 1241–1299.

Dalley, G. 1988. *Ideologies of caring: rethinking community and collectivism. Women in society.* Houndmills, Basingstoke: Macmillan Education.

Daniels, N. 2010. 'Capabilities, opportunity, and health'. In H. Brighouse and I. Robeyns (eds) *Measuring justice: primary goods and capabilities.* Cambridge: Cambridge University Press, pp. 131–149.

Davidson, L. and Roe, D. 2007. 'Recovery from versus recovery in serious mental illness: one strategy for lessening confusion plaguing recovery'. *Journal of Mental Health* 16 (4): 459–470.

Davidson, L. *et al.* 2001. '"Simply to be let in": inclusion as a basis for recovery'. *Psychiatric Rehabilitation Journal* 24 (4): 375–388.

Davidson, L. *et al.* 2005. 'Processes of recovery in serious mental illness: findings from a multinational study'. *American Journal of Psychiatric Rehabilitation* 8 (3): 177–201.

Davidson, L. *et al.* 2009. 'A capabilities approach to mental health transformation: a conceptual framework for the recovery era'. *Canadian Journal of Community Mental Health (Revue canadienne de santé mentale communautaire)* 28 (2): 35–46.

Davidson, L., Rakfeldt, J. and Strauss, J. 2011. *The roots of the recovery movement in psychiatry: lessons learned.* Chichester: Wiley-Blackwell.

Deegan, P.E. 1988. 'Recovery: the lived experience of rehabilitation'. *Psychosocial Rehabilitation Journal* 11 (4): 11–19.

Deegan, P.E. 1996a. 'Recovery and the conspiracy of hope'. Online. Available at https://link.springer.com/chapter/10.1007/978-3-319-28616-7_9 (accessed 5 March 2017).

Deegan, P.E. 1996b. 'Recovery as a journey of the heart'. *Psychiatric Rehabilitation Journal* 19 (3): 91–97.

Deegan, P.E. and Drake, R. 2006. 'Shared decision-making and medication management in the recovery process'. *Psychiatric Services* 57 (11): 1636–1639.

Deneulin, S. 2008. 'Beyond individual freedom and agency: structures of living together in the capability approach'. In F. Comim, M. Qizilbash and S. Alkire (eds) *The capability approach: concepts, measures and applications*. Cambridge: Cambridge University Press, pp. 105–124.

Department of Health. 2001. *The journey to recovery: the government's vision for mental health care*. London: Department of Health.

Department of Health. 2005. *Delivering race equality in mental health care: an action plan for reform inside and outside services and the government's response to the Independent inquiry into the death of David Bennett*. London: Department of Health.

Department of Health. 2009. *New horizons: a shared vision for mental health*. London: Department of Health.

Department of Health. 2011. *No health without mental health: a cross-government mental health outcomes strategy for people of all ages*. London: HMSO.

DeVault, M.L. 1994. *Feeding the family: the social organization of caring as gendered work*. Chicago, IL: University of Chicago Press.

Dickson-Swift, V. *et al.* 2007. 'Doing sensitive research: what challenges do qualitative researchers face?' *Qualitative Research* 7 (3): 327–353.

Dickson-Swift, V. *et al.* 2008. 'Risk to researchers in qualitative research on sensitive topics: issues and strategies'. *Qualitative Health Research* 18 (1): 133–144.

Dobransky, K. 2011. 'Labeling, looping, and social control: contextualizing diagnosis in mental health care'. In P.J. McGann and D.J. Hutson (eds) *Sociology of diagnosis. Advances in medical sociology*, Vol. 12. Bingley: Emerald Publishing Group, pp. 111–131.

Dugsin, R. 2001. 'Conflict and healing in family experience of second-generation emigrants from India living in North America'. *Family Process* 40 (2): 233–241.

Edgley, A. *et al.* (2012) 'The politics of recovery in mental health: a left libertarian policy analysis'. *Social Theory and Health* 10 (2): 121–140.

Ehrenreich, B. 2010. *Smile or die: how positive thinking fooled America and the world.* London: Granta.

Elder, G.H., Johnson, M.K. and Crosnoe, R. 2003. 'The emergence and development of life course theory'. In J.T. Mortimer and M.J. Shanahan (eds) *Handbook of the life course*. New York: Springer, pp. 3–19.

Emslie, C. *et al.* 2006.'Men's accounts of depression: reconstructing or resisting hegemonic masculinity?' *Social science and medicine* 62 (9): 2246–2257.

Equality Act 2010 (c. 15). London: HMSO.

Evans, P. 2002. 'Collective capabilities, culture, and Amartya Sen's "development as freedom"'. *Studies in Comparative International Development* 37 (2): 54–60.

Faulkner, A. 2004. *The ethics of survivor research: Guidelines for the ethical conduct of research carried out by mental health service users and survivors*. Bristol: The Policy Press. Online. Available at www.jrf.org.uk/file/36008/download?token=fy32S63X (accessed 31 October 2016).

Fernando, S. 2002. *Mental health, race and culture*. 2nd edn. Basingstoke: Palgrave.

Fernando, S. 2003. *Cultural diversity, mental health and psychiatry: The struggle against racism*. Hove: Brunner-Routledge.

Fernando, S. 2006. 'Stigma, racism and power'. *Aotearoa Ethnic Network Journal* 1 (1): 24–28.

Fernando, S. 2009. 'Meanings and realities'. In S. Fernando and F. Keating (eds) *Mental health in a multi-ethnic society: a multidisciplinary handbook*. London: Routledge, pp. 13–26.

Ferns, P. 2005. *Chinese people don't take milk and love to eat jelly?* London: Social Perspectives Network. Online. Available at www.spn.org.uk/index.php?id=828 (accessed 19 September 2013).

Fountain, J. and Hicks, J. 2010. *Delivering race equality in mental health care: report on the findings and outcomes of the community engagement programme 2005–2008.* Preston: University of Central Lancashire. Online. Available at www.better-health. org.uk/resources/research/delivering-race-equality-mental-health-care-report-findings-and-outcomes-communit (accessed 31 October 2016).

Fraser, N. 1995. 'From redistribution to recognition? Dilemmas of justice in a "post-socialist" age'. *New Left Review* 212: 63–68.

Fulford, B. and Wallcraft, J. 2009. 'Values-based practice and service user involvement in mental health research'. In J. Wallcraft, B. Schrank, and M. Amering (eds) *Handbook of service user involvement in mental health research*. Chichester: John Wiley & Sons: 37–60.

George, L.K. 2007. 'Life course perspectives on social factors and mental illness'. In W.R. Avison, J. D. McLeod, and B.A. Pescosolido (eds) *Mental health, social mirror.* New York: Springer, pp. 191–218.

Gerhardt, U. 1979. 'The Parsonian paradigm and the identity of medical sociology'. *Sociological Review* 27 (2): 235–251.

Godderis, R. 2011. 'From talk to action: mapping the diagnostic process in psychiatry'. In P.J. McGann and D.J. Hutson (eds) *Sociology of diagnosis. Advances in medical sociology*, Vol. 12. Bingley: Emerald Publishing Group, pp. 133–152.

Goldberg *et al.*, 1997. 'The validity of two versions of the GHQ in the WHO study of mental illness in general health care'. *Psychological Medicine* 27 (1): 191–197.

Green, G. *et al.* 2002. 'Is the English National Health Service meeting the needs of mentally distressed Chinese women?' *Journal of Health Services Research and Policy* 7 (4): 216–221.

Green, G. *et al.* 2006. '"We are not completely Westernised": dual medical systems and pathways to health care among Chinese migrant women in England'. *Social Science and Medicine* 62 (6): 1498–1509.

Habermas, J. 1987. *Lifeworld and system: a critique of functionalist reason. Theory of communicative action*, Vol. 2. Boston, MA: Beacon Press.

Hamilton, S. 2009. 'Money'. In J. Wallcraft, B. Schrank, and M. Amering (eds) *Handbook of service user involvement in mental health research*. Chichester: John Wiley & Sons, pp. 213–226.

Hankivsky, O. and Cormier, R. 2011. 'Intersectionality and public policy: some lessons from existing models'. *Political Research Quarterly* 64 (1): 217–229.

Harding, S.G. 1998. *Is science multicultural?: postcolonialisms, feminisms, and epistemologies.* Bloomington, IN: Indiana University Press.

Harley, C.R. and Mortimer, J.T. 2000. 'Social status and mental health in young adulthood: the mediating role of the transition to adulthood'. Paper presented at the Biennial Meeting of the Society for Research on Adolescence, Chicago, IL.

Harper, D. and Speed, E. (2012). 'Uncovering recovery: the resistible rise of recovery and resilience'. *Studies in Social Justice*, 6 (1): 9–25.

Harrison, G. *et al.* 2001. 'Recovery from psychotic illness: a 15- and 25-year international follow-up study'. *British Journal of Psychiatry* 178 (6): 506–517.

Heinz, W.R. and Krüger, H. 2001. 'Life course: innovations and challenges for social research'. *Current Sociology* 49 (2): 29–45.

Higgs, P., Jones, I.R. and Scambler, G. 2004. 'Class as variable, class as generative mechanism: the importance of critical realism for the sociology of health inequalities'. In B. Carter and C. New (eds) *Making realism work: realist social theory and empirical research*. Critical Realism: Interventions. London: Routledge, pp. 83–99.

Hoge, S.K. *et al.* 1997. 'Perceptions of coercion in the admission of voluntary and involuntary psychiatric patients'. *International Journal of Law and Psychiatry* 20 (2): 167–181.

Holroyd, E. *et al.* 1997. '"Doing the month": an exploration of postpartum practices in Chinese women'. *Health Care for Women International* 18 (3): 301–313.

Hopper, K. 2007. 'Rethinking social recovery in schizophrenia: what a capabilities approach might offer'. *Social Science and Medicine* 65 (5): 868–879.

Hopper, K. 2009. *Reframing first breaks and early crisis: a capabilities-informed approach*. International Network Toward Alternatives and Recovery: Working Papers for the INTAR Conference. Online. Available at www.intar.org/files/INTAR2009-NYC-HopperReframingFirstBreaksAndEarlyCrisis-CapabilitiesInformedApproach.doc (accessed 31 October 2016).

Hornstein, G.A. 2009. *Agnes's jacket: a psychologist's search for the meanings of madness*. New York: Rodale.

Huang, S.L. and Spurgeon, A. 2006. 'The mental health of Chinese immigrants in Birmingham'. *Ethnicity and Health* 11 (4): 365–387.

Hydén, L. 1997. 'Illness and narrative'. *Sociology of Health and Illness* 19 (1): 48–69.

Ibrahim, S.S. 2006. 'From individual to collective capabilities: the capability approach as a conceptual framework for self-help'. *Journal of Human Development* 7 (3): 397–416.

Jackson, W.A. 2005. 'Capabilities, culture and social structure'. *Review of Social Economy* 63 (1): 101–124.

Jones, A. 1997. 'High psychiatric morbidity amongst Irish immigrants'. Unpublished PhD Thesis. The Open University.

Jones, L., Hardiman, E. and Carpenter, J. 2007 'Mental health recovery: a strengths-based approach to culturally relevant services for African Americans'. *Journal of Human Behaviour in the Social Environment* 15 (2): 251–269.

Jutel, A. 2011. 'Sociology of diagnosis: a preliminary review'. In P.J. McGann and D.J. Hutson (eds) *Sociology of diagnosis: advances in medical sociology*, Vol. 12. Bingley: Emerald Publishing Group, pp. 3–32.

Kagan, C. *et al.* 2011. *Experiences of forced labour among Chinese migrant workers*. London: Joseph Rowntree Foundation. Online. Available at www.jrf.org.uk/sites/files/jrf/Chinese-migrants-forced-labour-full.pdf (accessed 31 October 2016).

Kalathil, J. *et al.* 2011a. *Recovery and resilience: African, African-Caribbean and South Asian women's narratives of recovering from mental distress*. London: Mental Health Foundation. Online. Available at www.mentalhealth.org.uk/publications/recovery-and-resilience/ (accessed 31 October 2016).

Kalathil, L. *et al.* 2011b. *Dancing to our own tunes: reassessing black and minority ethnic mental health service user involvement. Reprint of the 2008 report with a review of work undertaken to take the recommendations forward*. London: National Service User Network. Online. Available at www.nsun.org.uk/assets/downloadableFiles/dtoots_report_reprint-oct-20112.pdf (Accessed 31 October 2016).

Kantola, J. and Squires, J. 2010. 'The new politics of equality'. In C. Hay (ed.) *New directions in political science: responding to the challenges of an interdependent world*. London: Palgrave Macmillan, pp. 88–108.

Karlsen, S., and Nazroo, J.Y. 2002. 'Agency and structure: the impact of ethnic identity and racism on the health of ethnic minority people'. *Sociology of Health & Illness* 24 (1): 1–20.

Khader, S.J. 2011. *Adaptive preferences and women's empowerment*. Oxford: Oxford University Press.

Khader, S.J. 2012. 'Must theorising about adaptive preferences deny women's agency?' *Journal of Applied Philosophy* 29 (4): 302–317.

Kirmayer, L.J. 2001. 'Cultural variations in the clinical presentation of depression and anxiety: implications for diagnosis and treatment'. *Journal of Clinical Psychiatry* 62 (13 suppl.): 22–30.

Kjosavik, D.J. 2011. 'Standpoints and intersections: towards an indigenist epistemology'. In D.J. Rycroft and S. Dasgupta (eds) *The politics of belonging in India: becoming Adivasi*. London: Routledge, pp. 119–135.

Kleinman, A. 1977 (1967). 'Depression, somatization and the "new cross-cultural psychiatry"'. *Social Science & Medicine* 11 (1): 3–9.

Kleinman, A. 1988. *The illness narratives: suffering, healing and the human condition*. New York: Basic Books.

Kleinman, A., Eisenberg, L. and Good, B. 1978 'Culture, illness, and care: clinical lessons from anthropologic and cross-cultural research'. *Annals of Internal Medicine* 88 (2): 251–258.

Kraepelin, E. 1919. *Dementia praecox and paraphrenia*. Edinburgh: Livingstone.

Kwok, J. 2013. 'Factors that influence the diagnoses of Asian Americans in mental health: an exploration'. *Perspectives in Psychiatric Care* 49(4): 288–292.

Lai, W. 1979. 'Ch'an metaphors: waves, water, mirror, lamp'. *Philosophy East and West* 29 (3): 243–253.

Lai Yin Association. 1999. *The health needs of Chinese women in Sheffield*. Sheffield: Lai Yin Association.

Landeen, J. *et al.* 2000. 'Hope, quality of life, and symptom severity in individuals with schizophrenia'. *Psychiatric Rehabilitation Journal* 23 (4): 364–369.

Lane, P., Tribe, R. and Hui, R. 2010. 'Intersectionality and the mental health of elderly Chinese women living in the UK'. *International journal of Migration, Health and Social Care* 6 (4): 34–41.

Lee, M. *et al.* 2002. 'Chinese migrant women and families in Britain'. *Women's Studies International Forum* 25 (6): 607–618.

Lee, S. and Kleinman, A. 2007. 'Are somatoform disorders changing with time? The case of neurasthenia in China'. *Psychosomatic Medicine* 69 (9): 846–849.

Leff, J. and Warner, R. 2006. *Social inclusion of people with mental illness*. Cambridge: Cambridge University Press.

Lester, H. and Gask, L. 2006. 'Delivering medical care for patients with serious mental illness or promoting a collaborative model of recovery?' *British Journal of Psychiatry* 188 (5): 4012–4402.

Lewis, L. 2012. 'The capabilities approach, adult community learning and mental health'. *Community Development Journal* 47 (4): 522–537.

Li, D. 1991. 'The experience of psychiatrists managing Chinese patients in Merseyside'. *Psychiatric Bulletin* 15 (12): 727–728.

Li, P.L. and Logan, S. 1999. *The mental health needs of Chinese people in England: a report of a national survey*. London: Chinese National Healthy Living Centre.

McCall, L. 2005. 'The complexity of intersectionality'. *Signs* 30 (3): 1771–1800.

McKenzie, K., Whitley, R. and Weich, S. 2002. 'Social capital and mental health'. *British Journal of Psychiatry* 181 (4): 280–283.

Marmot, M. *et al.* 2010. *Fair society, healthy lives: The Marmot Review*. Online. Available at www.instituteofhealthequity.org/projects/fair-society-healthy-lives-the-marmot-review (accessed 31 October 2016).

Mattheys, K. 2015. 'The coalition, austerity and mental health'. *Disability & Society* 30(3): 475–478.

Menzies, R.J., Reaume, G. and LeFrançois, B.A. (eds) 2013. *Mad matters: a critical reader in Canadian mad studies.* Toronto, ON: Canadian Scholars' Press.

Mezzina, R. *et al.* 2006. 'The social nature of recovery: discussion and implications for practice'. *American Journal of Psychiatric Rehabilitation* 9 (1): 63–80.

Mills, C. Wright. 2000. *The sociological imagination*. Oxford: Oxford University Press.

Mitra, S. 2006. 'The capability approach and disability'. *Journal of Disability Policy Studies* 16 (4): 236–247.

Morgan, C. *et al.* 2004. 'Negative pathways to psychiatric care and ethnicity: the bridge between social science and psychiatry'. *Social Science & Medicine* 58 (4): 739–752.

Morrow, M. 2013. 'Recovery: progressive paradigm or neoliberal smokescreen?' In R.J. Menzies, G. Reaume and B.A. LeFrançois (eds) *Mad matters: a critical reader in Canadian mad studies.* Toronto, ON: Canadian Scholars' Press, pp. 323–333.

Morrow, M. and Weisser, J. 2012. 'Towards a social justice framework of mental health recovery'. *Studies in Social Justice* 6 (1): 27–43.

Nazroo, J.Y. 1997. *Ethnicity and mental health: findings from a national community survey.* London: Policy Studies Institute

Nazroo, J.Y. 1998. 'Genetic, cultural or socio-economic vulnerability? Explaining ethnic inequalities in health'. *Sociology of Health & Illness* 20 (5): 710–730.

Nazroo, J.Y. 2003. 'The structuring of ethnic inequalities in health: economic position, racial discrimination, and racism'. *American Journal of Public Health* 93 (2): 277–284.

British Academy (ed.). 2014. '*If you could do one thing . . .*': nine local actions to reduce health inequalities. London: British Academy,

Nussbaum, M.C. 2000. *Women and human development: the capabilities approach.* Cambridge: Cambridge University Press.

Oliver, P. 2006. 'Purposive sampling'. In V. Jupp (ed.) *The SAGE dictionary of social research methods.* London: Sage. Online. Available at http://srmo.sagepub.com/view/the-sage-dictionary-of-social-research-methods/n162.xml (accessed 31 October 2016).

Onken, S.J. *et al.* 2002. *Mental health recovery: what helps and what hinders? A national research project for the development of recovery facilitating system performance indicators.* Alexandria, VA: National Technical Assistance Center for State Mental Health Planning.

Orton, M. 2011. 'Flourishing lives: the capabilities approach as a framework for new thinking about employment, work and welfare in the 21st century'. *Work, Employment & Society* 25 (2): 352–360.

Pang, M. 1999. 'The employment situation of young Chinese adults in the British labour market'. *Personnel Review* 28 (1/2): 41–57.

Parken, A. and Young, H. 2008. *Facilitating cross-strand working.* Cardiff: Equality and Human Rights Commission. Online. Available at www.scie-socialcareonline.org.uk/facilitating-cross-strand-working/r/a11G00000017xqDIAQ (accessed 31 October 2016).

Parker, D. 1995. *Through different eyes: the cultural identity of young Chinese people in Britain.* Aldershot: Avebury.

Parker, D. and Song, M. 2007. 'Inclusion, participation and the emergence of British Chinese websites'. *Journal of Ethnic and Migration Studies* 33 (7): 1043–1061.

Parker, I. *et al.* 1997. *Deconstructing psychopathology.* London: Sage.

Parr, H. 1997. 'Mental health, public space, and the city: questions of individual and collective access'. *Environment and Planning D: Society and Space* 15 (4): 435–454.

Parse, R. R. 1999. *Hope: an international human becoming perspective.* Sudbury, MA: Jones & Bartlett.

Parsons, T. (1975). 'The sick role and the role of the physician reconsidered'. *The Milbank Memorial Fund Quarterly. Health and Society*, 257–278.

Pendleton, D.A. and Bochner, S. 1980. 'The communication of medical information in general practice consultations as a function of patients' social class'. *Social Science & Medicine. Part A: Medical Psychology & Medical Sociology* 14 (6): 669–673.

Perlin, M.L. 1992. 'On "sanism"'. *Southern Methodist University Law Review* 46: 373–407.

Perlin, M.L. 1999. 'Half-wracked prejudice leaped forth: sanism, pretextuality, and why and how mental disability law developed as it did'. *Journal of Contemporary Legal Issues* 10 (3): 3–36. Online. Available at http://heinonline.org/HOL/LandingPage?collection=journals&handle=hein.journals/contli10&div=5&id=&page= (accessed 31 October 2016).

Perlin, M.L. 2000. *The hidden prejudice: mental disability on trial.* Washington, DC: American Psychological Association.

Pescosolido, B.A., Gardner, C.B. and Lubell, K.M. 1998. 'How people get into mental health services: stories of choice, coercion and "muddling through" from "first-timers"'. *Social Science & Medicine* 46 (2): 275–286.

Pharoah, R. and Lau, S. 2009. *Shaping the future for London's Chinese community: a research based policy briefing.* London: Chinese in Britain Forum. Online. Available at www.chinesemigration.org.uk/download/MigrationBriefing.pdf (accessed 31 October 2016).

Pilgrim, D. 2008. '"Recovery" and current mental health policy'. *Chronic Illness* 4 (4): 295–304.

Pilgrim, D. 2013. 'The failure of diagnostic psychiatry and some prospects of scientific progress offered by critical realism'. *Journal of Critical Realism* 12 (3): 336–358.

Pilgrim, D. 2014. 'Some implications of critical realism for mental health research'. *Social Theory & Health* 12(1): 1–21.

Pilgrim, D. 2015. *Understanding mental health: a critical realist exploration.* Abingdon: Routledge.

Pilgrim, D. 2016.'Peter Sedgwick, proto-critical realist?' *Critical and Radical Social Work.* https://doi.org/10.1332/204986016X14651166264390.

Pilgrim, D. and Bentall, R. 1999. 'The medicalisation of misery: a critical realist analysis of the concept of depression'. *Journal of Mental Health* 8 (3): 261–274.

Pilgrim, D. and McCranie, A. 2013. *Recovery and mental health: a critical sociological account.* London: Palgrave Macmillan.

Pilgrim, D. and Tomasini, F. 2012. 'On being unreasonable in modern society: are mental health problems special?' *Disability & Society* 27(5): 631–646.

Poole, J.M. *et al.* 2012. 'Sanism, "mental health", and social work/education: a review and call to action'. *Intersectionalities: A Global Journal of Social Work Analysis, Research, Polity and Practice* 1: 20–36.

Portes, A. 1998. 'Social capital: its origins and applications in modern sociology'. *Annual Review of Sociology* 24: 1–24.

Powell, M. 2000. 'New Labour and the third way in the British welfare state: a new and distinctive approach?' *Critical Social Policy* 20 (1): 39–60.

Prilleltensky, I. (2005). 'Promoting well-being: time for a paradigm shift in health and human services'. *Scandinavian Journal of Public Health* 33 (66 suppl.): 53–60.

Ramon, S. *et al.* 2009. 'The rediscovered concept of recovery in mental illness'. *International Journal of Mental Health* 38 (2): 106–126.

Ramon, S., Healy, B. and Renouf, N., 2007. 'Recovery from mental illness as an emergent concept and practice in Australia and the UK'. *International Journal of Social Psychiatry* 53(2): 108–122.

Rapp, C.A. 1998. *The strengths model: case management with people suffering from severe and persistent mental illness*. Oxford: Oxford University Press.

Ratcliffe, P. 2004. *'Race', ethnicity and difference: imagining the inclusive society*. Maidenhead: McGraw-Hill International.

Ratcliff, P. 2012. '"Community cohesion": reflections on a flawed paradigm'. *Critical Social Policy* 32 (2): 262–281.

Read, J. 2010. 'Can poverty drive you mad? "Schizophrenia", socio-economic status and the case for primary prevention'. *New Zealand Journal of Psychology* 39(2): 7–19.

Read, J. and Bentall, R. P. 2012. 'Negative childhood experiences and mental health: theoretical, clinical and primary prevention implications'. *The British Journal of Psychiatry* 200 (2): 89–91.

Read, J. *et al.* 2006. 'Prejudice and schizophrenia: a review of the "mental illness is an illness like any other" approach'. *Acta Psychiatrica Scandinavica* 114 (5): 303–318.

Recovery in the Bin. 2016. 'The unrecovery star'. *Asylum Magazine* 23 (3): 18.

Repper, J. and Perkins, R. 2003. *Social inclusion and recovery: a model for mental health practice*. Edinburgh: Baillière Tindall.

Ridgway, P. 2001. 'ReStorying psychiatric disability: learning from first person recovery narratives'. *Psychiatric Rehabilitation Journal* 24 (4): 335–343.

Roberts, G.A. 2000. 'Narrative and severe mental illness: what place do stories have in an evidence-based world?' *Advances in Psychiatric Treatment* 6 (6): 432–441.

Robeyns, I. 2003. 'Is Nancy Fraser's critique of theories of distributive justice justified?' *Constellations* 10 (4): 538–554.

Robeyns, I. 2005. 'The capability approach: a theoretical survey'. *Journal of Human Development and Capabilities* 6 (1): 93–117.

Rochelle, T. L. and Shardlow, S. M. 2014. 'Health, functioning and social engagement among the UK Chinese'. *International Journal of Intercultural Relations* 38: 142–150.

Rogers, A. and Pilgrim, D. 2010. *A sociology of mental health and illness*. 4th edn. Maidenhead: McGraw-Hill.

Rose, D. 2001. *Users' voices: the perspectives of mental health service users on community and hospital care*. London: Sainsbury Centre for Mental Health. Online. Available at www.scie-socialcareonline.org.uk/users—voices-the-perspectives-of-mental-health-service-users-on-community-and-hospital-care/r/a11G00000017rmWIAQ (accessed 30 October 2016).

Rose, D. 2009. 'Survivor-produced knowledge'. In A. Sweeney *et al.* (eds) *This is survivor research*. Ross-on-Wye: PCCS Books, pp. 38–43.

Rose, D. 2014. 'The mainstreaming of recovery'. *Journal of Mental Health* 23 (5): 217–218.

Ruger, J.P. 2009. *Health and social justice*. Oxford: Oxford University Press.

Russinova, Z. 1999. 'Providers' hope-inspiring competence as a factor optimizing psychiatric rehabilitation outcomes'. *Journal of Rehabilitation* 65 (4): 50–57.

Russo, J. and Sweeney, A. 2016. *Searching for a rose garden: challenging psychiatry, fostering mad studies*. Monmouth: PCCS Books.

Sacchetto, B. *et al.* 2016. 'The capabilities questionnaire for the community mental health context (CQ-CMH): a measure inspired by the capabilities approach and constructed through consumer–researcher collaboration'. *Psychiatric Rehabilitation Journal* 39 (1): 55–61.

Salaff, J. 1981. *Working daughters of Hong Kong: filial piety or power in the family?* Cambridge: Cambridge University Press.

Saleeby, P.W. 2007. 'Applications of a capability approach to disability and the International Classification of Functioning, Disability and Health (ICF) in social work practice'. *Journal of Social Work in Disability & Rehabilitation* 6 (1–2): 217–232.

Salway, S.M. *et al.* 2010. *Fair society, healthy lives: a missed opportunity to address ethnic inequalities in health.* London: British Medical Journal. Online. Available at www.bmj.com/rapid-response/2011/11/02/fair-society-healthy-lives-missed-opportunity-address-ethnic-inequalities- (accessed 31 October 2016).

Sayer, A. 1992. *Method in social science: a realist approach.* London: Routledge.

Sayer, A. 1999. 'On not reducing the systemworld to the lifeworld'. *European Urban and Regional Studies* 6 (4): 319–322.

Sayer, A. 2012. 'Capabilities, contributive injustice and unequal divisions of labour'. *Journal of Human Development and Capabilities* 13 (4): 580–596.

Scambler, G. 2002. *Health and social change: a critical theory.* Buckingham: Open University Press.

Scheff, T.J. 1966. *Being mentally ill: a sociological theory.* Chicago, IL: Chicago University Press.

Scottish Recovery Network. 2008. *Finding strengths from within.* Edinburgh: Health Scotland.

Sedgwick, P. 1982. *Psycho politics: Laing, Foucault, Goffman, Szasz, and the future of mass psychiatry.* New York: Harper & Row.

Semmler, P.L. and Williams, C.B. 2000. 'Narrative therapy: a storied context for multicultural counseling'. *Journal of Multicultural Counseling and Development* 28 (1): 51–62.

Sen, A. 1984. 'Rights and capabilities'. In Sen, A., *Resources, values and development.* Oxford: Basil Blackwell, pp. 307–325.

Sen, A. 1997. 'Inequality, unemployment and contemporary Europe'. *International Labour Review* 136: 155.

Sen, A. 1999. *Development as freedom.* Oxford: Oxford University Press.

Sen, A. 2000. *Social exclusion: concept, application, and scrutiny.* Social Development Papers No. 1. Manila: Asian Development Bank. Online. Available at www.adb.org/sites/default/files/publication/29778/social-exclusion.pdf (accessed 31 October 2016).

Shakespeare, T. 2007. 'Disability rights and wrongs'. *Scandinavian Journal of Disability Research* 9 (3): 278–281.

Shanahan, M. J. 2000. 'Pathways to adulthood in changing societies: variability and mechanisms in life course perspective'. *Annual Review of Sociology* 26: 667–692.

Shiner, M. *et al.* 2009. 'When things fall apart: gender and suicide across the life-course'. *Social Science & Medicine* 69 (5): 738–746.

Simpson, L. *et al.* 2006. *Ethnic minority populations and the labour market: an analysis of the 1991 and 2001 Census.* No. 333. Leeds: Corporate Document Services.

Slade, M. *et al.* 2012. 'International differences in understanding recovery: systematic review'. *Epidemiology and Psychiatric Sciences* 21 (4): 353–364.

Social Perspectives Network. 2007. *Whose recovery is it anyway?* Paper 11. Online. Available at http://spn.org.uk/wp-content/uploads/2015/02/Recovery_and_Diversity_Booklet.pdf (accessed 31 October 2016).

Southside Partnership/Fanon. 2008. *Report of the community led research project focussing on male African and African Caribbean perspectives on recovery.* London: NIMHE.

Spandler, H., Anderson, J. and Sapey, B. (eds) 2015. *Madness, distress and the politics of disablement.* Bristol: Policy Press.

Spandler, H. and Calton, T. 2009. 'Psychosis and human rights: conflicts in mental health policy and practice'. *Social Policy & Society* 8 (2): 245–256.

Sproston, K. and Mindell, J. (eds) 2006. *Health survey for England, 2004. Vol. 1: the health of minority ethnic groups*. Leeds: Information Centre.

Steensen, J.J. 2006. 'Biographical interviews in a critical realist perspective'. Paper presented at the IACR Annual Conference 2006, University of Tromsø.

Straughan, H. 2009. 'Influencing change: user or researcher? Elitism in research'. In A. Sweeney *et al.* (eds) *This is survivor research*. Ross-on-Wye: PCCS Books, pp. 107–119.

Szasz, T.S. 1961. *The myth of mental illness: foundations of a theory of personal conduct*. New York: Harper & Row.

Szasz, T.S. 1971. 'The sane slave: a historic note on the use of medical diagnosis as justificatory rhetoric'. *American Journal of Psychotherapy* 25 (2): 228–239.

Tang, L. 2016. 'Barriers to recovery for Chinese mental health service-users in the UK: a case for community development'. *Community Development Journal*. doi: 10.1093/cdj/bsw025.

Tang, L. Forthcoming. 'Community development and Chinese mental health service users in the UK'. In G. Craig (ed.) *Community organising against racism: 'race', ethnicity and community development*. Bristol: Policy Press.

Taylor, R.E. 2001. 'Death of neurasthenia and its psychological reincarnation: a study of neurasthenia at the National Hospital for the Relief and Cure of the Paralysed and Epileptic, Queen Square, London, 1870–1932'. *British Journal of Psychiatry* 179 (6): 550–557.

Tew, J. *et al.* 2012. 'Social factors and recovery from mental health difficulties: a review of the evidence'. *British Journal of Social Work* 42 (3): 443–460.

Thích, N.H. 2010. *Peace is every step: the path of mindfulness in everyday life*. London: Rider.

Thomas, C. 2008. 'Disability: getting it "right"'. *Journal of Medical Ethics* 34 (1): 15–17.

Thornicroft, G., Rose, D. and Kassam, A. 2007. 'Discrimination in health care against people with mental illness'. *International Review of Psychiatry* 19 (2): 113–122.

Thornicroft, G., *et al.* 2007. 'Stigma: ignorance, prejudice or discrimination?' *British Journal of Psychiatry* 190 (3): 192–193.

Tong, Y. *et al.* 2014. *The Chinese population in North East England*. Durham: North East Race Crime and Justice Regional Research Network.

Tran, L. *et al.* 2008. *Report of the community led research project focussing on the mental health service needs of Chinese elders in Westminster, Kensington and Chelsea and Brent*. London: The Chinese National Healthy Living Centre. Online. Available at www.cnhlc.org.uk/pdf/CommunityEngagement-Report.pdf (accessed 31 October 2016).

Tse, S. *et al.* 2012. 'Recovery in Hong Kong: service user participation in mental health services'. *International Review of Psychiatry* 24 (1): 40–47.

Unterhalter, E. 2009. 'Education'. In S. Denenulin and L. Shahani (eds) *An introduction to the human development and capability approach: freedom and agency*. London: Earthscan, pp. 207–227.

van Mens-Verhulst, J. and Radtke, L. 2008. *Intersectionality and mental health: a case study*. Online. Available at www.vanmens.info/verhulst/en/wp-content/INTERSECTIONALITY%20AND%20MENTAL%20HEALTH2.pdf (accessed 31 October 2016).

Viruell-Fuentes, E. A., Miranda, P. Y., and Abdulrahim, S. 2012. 'More than culture: structural racism, intersectionality theory, and immigrant health'. *Social Science & Medicine* 75 (12): 2099–2106.

Wadsworth, M.E.J. 1997. 'Health inequalities in the life course perspective'. *Social Science & Medicine* 44 (6): 859–869.

Walby, S. 2007. 'Complexity theory, systems theory, and multiple intersecting social inequalities'. *Philosophy of the Social Sciences* 37 (4): 449–470.

Walby, S., Armstrong, J. and Strid, S. 2012. 'Intersectionality and the quality of the gender equality architecture'. *Social politics: International Studies in Gender, State & Society* 19 (4): 446–481.

Walker, M. 2006. *Higher education pedagogies [electronic resource]: a capabilities approach.* Maidenhead: McGraw-Hill International.

Wallcraft, J. 2001. 'Turning towards recovery? A study of personal narratives of mental health crisis and breakdown'. Unpublished PhD Thesis, London South Bank University.

Wallcraft, J. 2010. 'The capabilities approach in mental health: what are the implications for research and outcome measurement?' Paper presented at the Qualitative Research on Mental Health conference, University of Nottingham.

Wallcraft, J. 2011. 'Service users' perceptions of quality of life measurement in psychiatry'. *Advances in Psychiatric Treatment* 17 (4): 266–274.

Wallcraft, J. and Hopper, K. 2015. 'The capability approach and the social model of mental health. In H. Spandler, J. Anderson, and B. Sapey (eds) *Madness, distress and the politics of disablement.* Bristol: Policy Press, pp. 83–97.

Wallcraft, J. and Nettle, M. 2009. 'History, context and language'. In J. Wallcraft, B. Schrank, and M. Amering (eds) *Handbook of service user involvement in mental health research.* Chichester: John Wiley & Sons: 1–11.

Ware, N.C. *et al.* 2007. 'Connectedness and citizenship: redefining social integration'. *Psychiatric Services* 58 (4): 469–474.

Ware, N.C. *et al.* 2008. 'A theory of social integration as quality of life'. *Psychiatric Services* 59 (1): 27.

Warner, R. 1994. *Recovery from schizophrenia: psychiatry and political economy.* 2nd edn. London: Routledge.

Watters, C. 1996. 'Representations of Asian's mental health in psychiatry'. In C. Samson and N. South (eds) *The social construction of social policy: Methodologies, racism, citizenship and the environment.* London: MacMillan.

Weisser, J., Morrow, M. and Jamer, B. 2011. *A critical exploration of social inequities in the mental health recovery literature.* Vancouver, BC: Centre for the Study of Gender, Social Inequities and Mental Health (CGSM).

Welzel, C. and Inglehart, R. 2010. 'Agency, values, and well-being: a human development model'. *Social Indicators Research* 97 (1): 43–63.

Wheat, K. *et al.* 2010. 'Mental illness and the workplace: conceal or reveal?' *Journal of the Royal Society of Medicine* 103 (3): 83–86.

Wilkinson, R.G. and Pickett, K. 2011. *The spirit level.* New York: Bloomsbury Press.

Williams, G.H. 2003. 'The determinants of health: structure, context and agency'. *Sociology of Health & Illness* 25 (3): 131–154.

Williams, S.J. 1999. 'Is anybody there? Critical realism, chronic illness and the disability debate'. *Sociology of Health & Illness* 21 (6): 797–819.

Williams, S.J. 2000. 'Chronic illness as biographical disruption or biographical disruption as chronic illness? Reflections on a core concept'. *Sociology of Health & Illness* 22 (1): 40–67.

Williams, S.J. 2003. 'Beyond meaning, discourse and the empirical world: critical realist reflections on health'. *Social Theory & Health* 1 (1): 42–71.

Williams, S.J. 2005. 'Parsons revisited: from the sick role to . . . ?' *Health* 9 (2): 123–144.

Wong, G. and Cochrane, R. 1989. 'Generation and assimilation as predictors of psychological well-being in British-Chinese'. *Social Behaviour* 4 (1): 1–14.

Wong, Y.L. and Tsang, A.K.T. 2004. 'When Asian immigrant women speak: from mental health to strategies of being'. *American Journal of Orthopsychiatry* 74 (4): 456–466.

Wu, B., Guo, L. and Sheehan, J. 2010. *Employment conditions of Chinese migrant workers in the East Midlands: a pilot study in a context of economic recession.* Beijing: ILO. Online. Available at www.ilo.org/beijing/what-we-do/publications/WCMS_145878/lang—en/index.htm (accessed 31 October, 2016).

Wu, S.W. 2008. 'Xianggang gaodeng jiaoyu kuangzhan de jingli' [The process of expansion of higher education in Hong Kong] *Zhongzheng jiaoyu yanjiu* [*Chung Cheng Educational Studies*] 7 (1): 1–28.

Yanos, P.T. and Hopper, K. 2008. 'On "false, collusive objectification": becoming attuned to self-censorship, performance and interviewer biases in qualitative interviewing'. *International Journal of Social Research Methodology* 11 (3): 229–237.

Yanos, P.T., Knight, E.L. and Roe, D. 2007. 'Recognizing a role for structure and agency: integrating sociological perspectives into the study of recovery from severe mental illness'. In W.R. Avison, J.D. McLeod and B.A. Pescosolido (eds) *Mental health, social mirror.* New York: Springer, pp. 407–433.

Yanos, P.T., Roe, D. and Lysaker, P.H. (2010). 'The impact of illness identity on recovery from severe mental illness'. *American Journal of Psychiatric Rehabilitation* 13 (2): 73–93.

Yeung, E.Y.W. *et al.* 2012. 'Role of social networks in the help-seeking experiences among Chinese suffering from severe mental illness in England: a qualitative study'. *British Journal of Social Work* 43 (3): 486–503.

Yeung, E.Y.W. *et al.* 2015 'Satisfaction with social care: the experiences of people from Chinese backgrounds with physical disabilities', *Health & Social Care in the Community* 24 (6): e101–e200.

Yip, K.S. 2005. 'Taoistic concepts of mental health: implications for social work practice with Chinese communities'. *Families in Society* 86 (1): 35–46.

Yu, W.K. 2000. *Chinese older people: A need for social inclusion in two communities.* Bristol: The Policy Press.

Yu, W.K.S. 2006. 'Adaptation and tradition in the pursuit of good health Chinese people in the UK: the implications for ethnic-sensitive social work practice'. *International Social Work* 49 (6): 757–766.

Zimmermann, B. 2006. 'Pragmatism and the capability approach challenges in social theory and empirical research'. *European Journal of Social Theory* 9 (4): 467–484.

Index